## TABLE OF

# Top 20 Test Taking Tips

1. Carefully follow all the test registration procedures
2. Know the test directions, duration, topics, question types, how many questions
3. Setup a flexible study schedule at least 3-4 weeks before test day
4. Study during the time of day you are most alert, relaxed, and stress free
5. Maximize your learning style; visual learner use visual study aids, auditory learner use auditory study aids
6. Focus on your weakest knowledge base
7. Find a study partner to review with and help clarify questions
8. Practice, practice, practice
9. Get a good night's sleep; don't try to cram the night before the test
10. Eat a well balanced meal
11. Know the exact physical location of the testing site; drive the route to the site prior to test day
12. Bring a set of ear plugs; the testing center could be noisy
13. Wear comfortable, loose fitting, layered clothing to the testing center; prepare for it to be either cold or hot during the test
14. Bring at least 2 current forms of ID to the testing center
15. Arrive to the test early; be prepared to wait and be patient
16. Eliminate the obviously wrong answer choices, then guess the first remaining choice
17. Pace yourself; don't rush, but keep working and move on if you get stuck
18. Maintain a positive attitude even if the test is going poorly
19. Keep your first answer unless you are positive it is wrong
20. Check your work, don't make a careless mistake

**CPU**

The central processing unit, or CPU, receives information, processes it, and provides output. The CPU contains an arithmetic/logic unit (ALU) that performs mathematical operations including evaluating one piece of data against another piece of data. The control unit accesses input from the computer and determines its meaning in the instruction cycle. The control unit then accesses the required information needed to perform the request and provide output in the execution cycle. During CPU processing, information is held within registers. Input is stored in the instruction and address registers and once accessed from primary memory the output is stored in the storage register. The accumulator holds the output. CPU's vary in speed. Task completion is measured by the clock rate; the larger the word length a CPU can process, the faster it will be. Reduced instruction-set computing allows CPU's containing the technology to perform functions in a single cycle, making them faster.

**Primary storage**

Binary numbers are applied to all data input that is stored in the primary storage area of a computer. Silicon chips hold the data and the number of chips can be increased so the computer will hold more memory. Memory that can be accessed by the computer but cannot be added to, or changed, is called read only memory. The memory is nonvolatile or constant regardless of whether or not the computer is receiving power. Volatile memory, in contrast, is lost if there is no power to the computer. Random access memory is volatile and is where memory is stored that is used to run programs. The memory can be accessed randomly which means the computer does not have to process through an order to obtain the information. Cache memory is short-term memory that can be accessed more quickly than random access memory.

**Secondary storage**

Secondary storage is a unit where memory can be stored apart from the computer unit and without the use of primary storage. Magnetic tapes have been used to store data. Much like a cassette tape, memory is stored on reels of tape. Magnetic tapes are inexpensive but the data stored on the tapes cannot be accessed directly. If information that is stored halfway through the tape needs to be accessed, the tape has to be played to that point. Magnetic disks, both hard and floppy, are used as secondary storage devices. The disks have rings that store information in sectors and tracks. Information can be accessed directly from a part of the disk. Optical disks or compact disks store memory in laser created divots imprinted on the plastic disk. Some disks are read only, so the information can be accessed from the disk, but once the disk is full, no more can be added. Some disks are rewritable so information can be changed and the disk can be rewritten. DVD's can store information on the front and back of the disk and can often hold more information than CD's.

## Magneto-optical disks, optical cards, and smart cards

Sometimes it is necessary for users to be able to access a large amount of stored data at the same time. Magneto-optical disks make this possible, because they are small optical devices that can be stored together in a larger optical jukebox storage system. The disks allow information to be added and removed from their magnetic rings produced by lasers. Optical cards, sometimes called laser cards, are little cards where information can be stored. The size of the memory constitutes how much information can be stored on each card; once stored, the information cannot be removed. Smart cards differ from optical cards in that they can store and process some information. Smart cards can be used by healthcare providers to access a patient's records, including insurance information. Patients can store money on the smart card, much like a savings account to cover healthcare related costs.

## Input devices

Keyboards are the most-used type of computer input unit. The keyboard contains the letters of the alphabet and the numbers 0-9. The use of the characters allows the user to input required information into the computer system and the speed at which the user can type will determine how fast the information can be input. Computer input can be submitted by use of a pointing device like a mouse or touch screen. A mouse has a ball which can be moved around by the user to access computer menus. The mouse has buttons, typically right and left, which can be pressed to highlight information or bring up computer menus. Touch screens allow the user to physically touch where on the screen it wants the computer to access. Rather than double clicking an icon to open it with a mouse, the user can tap the screen twice to open the same icon. Global positioning systems and ATM machines both use touch screen technology.

Scanners are input devices that can read text and graphics. Barcode scanners are frequently used in the healthcare industry. A barcode is a series of parallel lines that contain information such as prescription or laboratory information. Optical mark readers are input devices that can read how a person marks answers to multiple-choice questions, often used to evaluate the quality of the patient's experience. Document scanners change input, including text and pictures, into pixels that the computer can understand. The documents can then be stored and accessed by the computer. Another type of input device is a handwriting-recognition device that can determine a user's information based on writing letters rather than typing. Voice input, or technology that can listen and interpret a persons language input, is available. Critics of the technology claim that the input devices do not understand all voice input correctly and do not understand different dialects and speech patterns.

**Output devices**

Video display terminals or computer monitors are the most common type of output unit and vary in screen size and resolution. The number of pixels displayed constitutes the quality of resolution. Video display terminals are rather large. Liquid crystal display monitors are flat screens, which use fluorescent light and crystal cells to present the computer's output. The flat monitor makes them more compact so they take up less room. Printed output is accessed through various printers including dot-matrix, inkjet, and laser printers. Dot-matrix printers use pins that hit a ribbon making a mark on a piece of paper. Inkjet printers use ink cartridges, which can be black or color rather than ribbons, to make marks on a page. Laser printers can produce high quality output and use memory to store information. The amount of memory capability the printer has directly relates to the quality of the output. Lasers control where the toner--which acts like ink--is placed on a paper. Portable printers are available for those individuals who need to print while away from the office.

**Classes of computers**

Supercomputers are computers that contain extremely quick processors and can use multiple processors in a parallel-processing configuration to achieve an objective. The healthcare industry typically uses mainframe computers to manage the abundant amount of information required. Shared-processing configurations control the processors in mainframe computers. Central processing units are bundled within close proximity known as processor clusters to share the responsibility of processing large amounts of information. Front-end processors help the main central processing unit by performing particular duties or helping with general functions. Smaller healthcare providers can use minicomputers to process their information. Minicomputers can be used alone or to support a mainframe computer system. Workstations are highly efficient microcomputers that can be used when something better than a microcomputer is required. Radiology imaging units are workstations that contain a large amount of storage space and are used to access and maintain x-rays. A personal computer is a term used interchangeably with microcomputer. These computers are easy to manage and relatively inexpensive and many can support a company's processing needs. Personal computers vary in size from a standard desktop computer, to a laptop, to a small personal blackberry device.

**General-purpose software**

General-purpose software is a type of application software which includes programs that can process a collection of data. Word processors are one type of general-purpose software that can adapt typed-in data including words. Word processing programs can make changes in grammar and spelling and can modify text based on the users' preferences. Desktop-publishing software is more advanced than word processing programs in the type of styles that can be applied to text. The software is ideal when pictures and graphics are needed in a page layout. Spreadsheet software provides users with a way to manage and manipulate large sets of numbers. The spreadsheet contains rows and columns made up of cells where data can be input. Preset formulas can perform basic functions such as addition and subtraction or the user can create more complex and unique formulas to perform complicated arithmetic functions. The cells to which the formulas will be applied must be selected by the user and the selection must be changed as data is added to the spreadsheet. The healthcare industry uses spreadsheets to evaluate costs and track patient care.

Statistical software is used to analyze input from the user by applying statistical methods to the data. The user must know the various statistical measurements to determine which type is best used to evaluate a problem. The software will perform the requested task but the user has to be able to interpret the output. Database-management software is software that allows the user to create access and manipulate a variety of databases, or collections of information. Users can compare information contained in databases. Presentation graphics software allows the user to create presentations with slides containing text and graphics. The visual displays produced can be used in meetings or training sessions to help the audience follow along with the information provided. Simulation software, such as MedModel for the healthcare industry, creates an image of the information that needs to be analyzed so the user can experiment with the data without changing the original data. Integrated software programs are programs that provide a variety of software programs in one package.

**Application-specific software**

Application-specific software is program software that healthcare organizations use to perform a specific function like filling out forms. Some of the software can be altered and used for a designated task that the purchaser needs completed and is specific to his or her organization. Other software is developed by the software company to complete tasks that most healthcare organizations need completed so the software is general and cannot be altered. Changing the software can be complicated and computer programmers have to be hired to complete the adaptations. Many healthcare managers do not have the time or resources available to make the adaptations, so many are opting to buy already developed software. Healthcare managers must be knowledgeable enough to understand the software they are purchasing, including knowing how many employees the system can handle, the price of potential upgrades to the program and how to maintain the privacy of the information input into the software.

**System-management software**

System-management software is designed to handle a computer's regularly scheduled functions. Operating systems are one type of system-management software that acts as an intermediary between the user and computer. The operating system designates what parts of the computer are required by the user when a task is requested. The user does not see the operating system at work but the operating system is responsible for communicating information to the user when something is not functioning properly. Most computers allow the user to multitask, or request the use of several applications at one time. The operating system has to allocate to the central processing unit which jobs need to be completed because the central processing unit cannot run more than one program simultaneously which is a process known as time-slicing. The user can give instructions to the operating system with text when the operating system interfacing is command-based. Icons are used to give the operating system commands when the operating system is graphically interfaced. Utility programs work to help the operating system and application programs. Utility programs aid normal computer functions like keeping records of newly created computer programs. Utility programs provide housekeeping on system files that are altered. When simple or difficult computing is required of the system, the utility programs handle the task.

## Programming language

Programming language is the language that the computer reads. All tasks requested of a computer have to be translated into a specific programming language that the computer recognizes. Each language is very detailed and precise and the language's organizational structure is called the syntax. The first programming language is known as machine language and requires the use of zeros and ones, which can be complicated for a programmer to learn. Abbreviations using letters was part of the second era of programming languages called assembly language. The codes are called mnemonics and are easier for the programmer to understand but an application is still required to change the mnemonics into number strings, or machine language, that the computer will understand. Determining the best mnemonics and memorizing the codes applied to each task is difficult for many programmers. Different fields of employment approach programming differently and mnemonics require a unified approach to computer programming.

Procedural, high-level languages describe the third era of programming language. The language is easier for the user to remember because it resembles user specific needs. The languages speak the language of the user rather than requiring the user to speak the language of the computer. For career fields that require the use of numbers and mathematics, the language FORTRAN is a popular choice and was the leader of the high-level languages. COBOL was the language developed that helped the business industry by providing a language that was similar to English. Much of the healthcare industry uses COBOL. ALGOL is a language that uses math and it with COBOL and FORTRAN were melded together to make a new language PL/1 which is intended to be used by all types of businesses formerly using the 3 separate languages. The healthcare industry frequently uses MUMPS, which is a program that gets information from a central place and can deliver it to several branches much like a tree. Pascal is a program designed for educational purposes of programming. C language is a language that is understood by multiple computers and therefore is popular.

The main difference between languages of the third and fourth era is that in the third era the programmer had to specifically tell the computer what it needed to do to perform a task. The programmer had to know the language and the system problem well enough to give detailed instructions. In fourth era programs, a problem can be input and the computer can translate the best course of action making these programming languages accessible to almost anyone. The future of computer languages involves the creation of strategies that will make a computer be able to understand any person's instructions and needs. The languages will need to be more user-friendly and voice recognition capabilities may be part of future programming languages. The computer will be able to understand and change natural language, or the user's language, into number sequences without the user ever having to input a programming language.

**Language translators**

Language translators change programming language into machine language, zeros and ones, so the computer will understand the commands. The language entered is called source code. Assemblers, compilers, interpreters and code-generation software are 4 kinds of language translators. Assemblers change mnemonics into binary codes and labels into addresses so the computer can understand the input assembly language. Compilers are designated for high-level programming languages because they translate multiple machine code directions. Source code provided by the organization is changed into object code the computer understands by compilers. The object code can then be used multiple times. If compilation is unnecessary because the program needs to be used infrequently, interpreters can be used instead. Interpreters translate language more quickly and can be altered frequently. Code-generation software translates code into third era languages, which provides a way for programmers who need code translated into language already established on their computer a quick alternative to writing it themselves.

**Network configurations**

A terminal-host system is a centralized system that uses a main computer to process information and perform all computing tasks. Several terminals can be connected to the main host terminal but their function is limited to data entry and answering questions requested of a software program. The terminals connected to the host computer can be located away from the host computer and the information input can be saved and sent to the host at a later time. It is easy to supervise the terminal-host system because the users cannot alter the host computer. Client/server computing systems allow the user more access to the system functions than in a terminal-host system. The clients are connected to an application server where they can access and edit information and the application server is connected to a data server which performs higher end functions, like managing databases. In a system based on file/server architecture, the server can be accessed by many network processors so the processing functions are shared by many terminals. A decentralized system where the computers do not have to access a central host computer is present in a peer network. The information on each can be shared and no main server is used.

## Transmission media

Within a network, information must be sent back and forth through the use of transmission media including metal wires and fiber-optic cables. Digital or analog transmission waves can be sent through electricity over metal wires such as copper. Unshielded twisted pair wires are the most frequently used copper wires and shielded twisted pair wires are used less frequently because they are more expensive and harder to work with. Coaxial cable is the most outdated type of copper cable. Electric current is changed to light, which is turned back into electric pulses through fiber-optic media. Single-mode fiber-optic cable is used for more complex networks because it can carry more data than multimode cable, a choice for smaller networks. Fiber-optic cable lasts longer, can carry information further, maintains more privacy, and has a greater bandwidth than copper cable. It is more difficult to work with than copper and costs more. Broadcast and radio media use radio waves to send information through the air. The information is less secure and can be easily interrupted by conflicting signals.

## Transmitters and receivers

For a high-speed LAN and microcomputer to communicate, a network interface card must be used to act as a translator for the 2 devices. Device drivers are downloaded onto the computer to make the communication possible. Copper-based and fiber optic modems alter signals sent between a transmitter and receiver so they can communicate. If a system requires a signal to go from analog to digital, a copper-based modem is used, but if the system requires a signal to go from digital to optical digital, fiber optic modems are used. A multiplexer can serve as an intermediary for many devices to one transmission line. Multiple networks can be joined by a bridge if their communication is equivalent. If the communication is not equivalent, a gateway can be used to join networks. At each gateway there is a router that dictates how information is shared on the network.

## Network components

If a network consists of computers sending and receiving messages to one main computer, a network controller must be present to guide the communication between the terminals and main computer. Local area networks use servers and detailed protocol to perform the function of network controllers. Mainframe computer systems use network control software to manage the network and monitor communication between the computers in the network. Network operating systems provide safeguards for both local and wide area networks. Network operating systems can either be a stand-alone computer system or can work along with the computer's regular operating system. Network software varies and price and usage needs should be weighed when deciding which software to chose.

## Physical topology networks

Computers send and receive information to outside equipment and the configuration necessary for the communication is referred to as physical topology. If some item like a wire or cable is used to connect the computer to outside equipment the item used is known as a bus. The communication of data back and forth between equipment is directed by a protocol known as Ethernet. When computers are linked together and information is sent from one to the next in an orbital fashion the network is known as a ring network. In a star network a main hub or concentrator acts as the central point where information is sent to and the hub determines where the information will be sent. Passive and active hubs simply send the messages to all of the connected devices, while intelligent hubs can determine where the information is supposed to be sent. When several types of networks are used together a hybrid network is developed.

## Electronic data interchange

Electronic data interchange, or EDI, is the term used to describe information sent back and forth between terminals without a person involved in the exchange. The exchange happens over different types of networks. The healthcare industry uses EDI for billing purposes and maintaining patient's personal information upon entering a facility. A patient's medical history is shared through EDI, including the conclusions of lab tests. The information has to be shared between the healthcare facility and the local health agency or the healthcare facility and hospital where the patient is admitted. Some companies offer software that oversees the supply-chain management of a healthcare organization, offering an alternative for hospital management who does not have the resources to employ a supply-chain manager. Wireless communication and the internet are 2 EDI mediums through which information is exchanged.

## Mobile computing

Many times healthcare providers do not have access to a desktop computer when visiting patients away from the office. Mobile computing is a type of technology that can be used to access and manipulate data away from an internet connection. A laptop or other mobile device is used but the information the user needs access to must be transferred to the mobile computer from the main computer before the information can be altered. As the user manipulates the data, it is not saved onto the main database until the user brings the computer back to the main computer and transfers the new data. Problems occur when more than one person is trying to access a patient's information. A doctor may give a patient a diagnosis away from the office and input the diagnosis via mobile computing. Before he or she transfers the diagnosis to the main database another specialist may have looked at the records and based a prescription on non-updated information. Mobile computing can cause major complications at times in the healthcare industry because information can change frequently.

## Spread spectrum, infrared and CDPD

Mobile computers like laptops and notebooks can be connected to the internet when away from the main computer with the use of wireless technology. 3 wireless topologies are spread spectrum, infrared, and Cellular Digital Packet Data. Through the use of an adapter card connecting to servers, wireless communication is achieved called spread spectrum. Spread spectrum uses radio frequencies to connect to the servers in a local area network. The healthcare industry uses spread spectrum technology commonly. Infrared technology is wireless, but has to be used in equipment that is close together. Wide area networks can use cell phone signals as a wireless signal which is technology called Cellular Digital Packet Data, or CDPD. CDPD is not as fast a regular connection but much more mobile. As CDPD network technology develops and gets a quicker connection rate it will become more popular because no phone line connection is necessary.

## Internet

An internet (non-capitalized) is created when several local area networks are linked together. The Internet (capitalized) is the biggest example of an internet where several networks connect to one main place which is a source of information for many millions of users. An Internet service provider gives companies, including healthcare organizations, access to the Internet for a price. The 2 types of connections Internet service providers offer are dial-up services and direct network connections. Dial-up services connect to the Internet through a phone connection or Integrated Services Digital Network (ISDN) line. The connection and the speed of the modem used will determine the quickness of the connection. An alternative to the use of a phone line to connect to the Internet is the use of direct network connections. Digital Subscriber Lines or cable modems are frequently used to make the connection between the computer and Internet service provider. Communication between the user and the Internet is administered by a program called the Transmission Control Protocol/Internet Protocol or TCP/IP.

The Internet is used in the healthcare setting in the areas if clinical and customer service applications, including providing patient access to medical information and conducting patient and physician interaction. Patients can access and view information regarding their own healthcare and view suggestions based on their health through web sites developed by insurance companies and medical providers. Patients use the Internet to find out about causes for their symptoms and treatments and bring what they have learned to their medical providers. As more physicians use the Internet, e-mail may become a communication medium between patients and their doctors. The more questions that can be answered via e-mail, the less time in the office a patient will take. Physicians should be accessing information on the Internet so they know what their clients are reading. Clinical applications such as benefit verification and treatment suggestions are being developed on the web, which creates a dynamic environment for real-time communication.

There are many concerns management must face and overcome as the Internet becomes the main communication tool in an organization. Privacy is the most important concern and needs to be protected. Protection can include the use of firewalls or putting information into code that people trying to illegally access the information cannot decipher. A home page is a common way for members within an organization to discuss and conduct business that is unique to their department. Home pages have to be monitored by management to make sure they are properly representing the organization as a whole. This oversight can include mandating certain visual displays that can be used on the department's home page. Management can implement a policy making it a requirement that they can review a home page before the home page or new information on an existing home page can be posted.

**Internet usage concerns**

Every healthcare organization has some policies, paperwork and procedures that are private and unique to their organization and the information must be legally withheld from public viewing. Information may be owned by its creator and therefore cannot be widely distributed by a healthcare organization. The Internet usage within an organization must be monitored so employees do not access inappropriate websites or accidentally create security risks to the system. E-mail must be strictly monitored by management to ensure that personal e-mails are not being viewed, downloaded and forwarded--all of which puts the organization at a great risk for viruses. It is the responsibility of management to ensure that employees are using e-mail appropriately and policies should be written to ensure employees know their expectations. Management must oversee the employees' use of the Internet to ensure over usage does not become a problem and that the Internet is used for business purposes rather than personal.

**Web site**

A web site is a page or pages of information which can be created by a person and accessed by anyone connecting to the Internet. A company can advertise, provide directions, and allow users to register, or provide any useful company information on a website. A browser is software that makes multiple pages that understand Hypertext Markup Language, or HTML possible. The person creating the web site names it by purchasing www address called a Uniform Resource Location, or URL. The URL can end in different domains including .org, .com, and .mil. A web server is used to save all of the information input to create the web site and the web pages are saved on the host computer. A server administrator reviews and updates the web site and several web pages, if applicable. Healthcare organizations will hire people within the company to create web sites or hire outside firms to create and maintain a website depending on the resources the organization has available.

**Intranet**

An intranet can be designed for use to send information back and forth within a company. An intranet is similar to the Internet in that it connects networks but a company's intranet is private and kept private because firewalls surround the information within the intranet. If there is a need to use a public network to send and receive information, the information can be protected through the use of a virtual private network, or VPN. A VPN protects both the customer and the service provider. The very use of an intranet can create security issues. People who want to access personal information try and discover ways to hack into or infiltrate a network. The network must be maintained for privacy and security and the healthcare industry is cautious of these privacy concerns. The intranet within the healthcare field is mainly informational, but as security technology increases, so will the intranet's use.

**Computer files**

The 2 types of computer files used to store information on computers are sequential computer files and direct-access computer files. Sequential computer files are tape drives that use fields, records and files to store information. A record holds basic information while a field provides memory for more detailed information about each record. A file holds and organizes the records according to the needs of the organization. In order to access or search the files, specific computer code had to be written because the information was sequential and could not be looked through or searched by any other means than manually. Direct-access storage devices, or DASD, were designed to make it possible to search and find a specific piece of information without manually reading through each file. The information on each file can be found because record numbers are applied to each file.

Program/file dependency is a problem because the program and file must be written in the same programming language for a computer to understand both. If multiple programs are necessary, compatibility becomes a problem unless all happen to be written in the same language, which is uncommon. Because computer systems in the healthcare industry have developed over time and there are many departments that handle patient information, requiring different computer programs that at times stand alone while at other times need to communicate, compatibility problems are difficult to overcome. The various healthcare programs are the admissions/discharge/transfer program, the order-entry and results-reporting program, the radiology program and the laboratory program. Data redundancy occurs when duplicate information is entered into the various programs that are designed to work together which uses unnecessary memory within the computer. Because people are needed to maintain files, time and money are wasted on redundant information. Data inconsistency becomes a problem when different information about the same person is entered into the system. The more data there is within the system, the higher the chance is for data inconsistencies.

**Databases**

Rather than using traditional computer files, databases can be created to store information. Data redundancy is reduced and data inconsistency can be maintained and eliminated by the database. Because a database fixes most of the problems related to data redundancy and inconsistency, the integrity of the data is strengthened. Through the use of a database, different departments can access and see information stored on the database. Privacy is better maintained because one central database can be protected rather than multiple file sources. The person controlling the database can apply rules that must be followed by anyone accessing the database. A central database provides a uniform source of information that is usable by all departments. The program and files are not dependent in a database and each can be accessed individually. The problems with databases surround the need for personnel to maintain the database which is much more complicated than traditional file systems. Databases can be expensive and less specific to the needs of each unit within an organization.
A hierarchal database model consists of branches leading from a main source. The equipment-maintenance database model uses a hierarchal database model. It consists of a department branching off to employees and equipment, and equipment branches off to technician and maintenance records. The main branch is referred to as a root and it can lead to several branches called child nodes. Child nodes become parent nodes when they branch off but each can only have a single parent node. A terminal node stands alone and has no other departments underneath it. The whole structure of a hierarchal database model is called a tree structure. Rather than a tree structure, a relational data model uses tables to organize information. Rows and columns are used to store single records and related information to each record. Because the database needs to be searchable, a key word is placed on all fields that can be found when necessary. A network data model is used when networks are used to hold information. Owners and members are words used to identify the branches in a network data model and they are joined by pointers, creating a set. Each member can have several owners so information is not repeated.

Hierarchal and network models have specific lines to which the branches are connected to each other. Information has to be sent from the main department to its subsequent branches in a line formation. The structure of the databases makes it difficult to search the databases because they are not specifically named. The healthcare industry typically uses hierarchal databases for large amounts of complicated information and relational databases for information that is easily input into a spreadsheet type of application like employee information. The relational database is the only database that can do ad hoc searches and because of its structure of rows and columns, many programs are compatible with it. A relational database is not as fast as the other 2 types of databases. Relational databases are best used when system oversight is required like in conservative applications. Relational databases are called for when decision-support applications are created because they need a database that is highly searchable.

**Data definition language**

A database has to be created and the information stored in the database must be explained and given meaning to, a process known as applying data defining language (DDL) to the database. Information stored on the computer is in bytes which are difficult for a person to understand and can be seen in the physical view of the computer. The logical view of the computer shows the person the same information but in more human terms because the information is quantified. The DDL converts the physical view into the logical view. To create a logical view, the user has to apply an explanation of each piece of information within the database called schema and subschema. Schema is created when 1 person needs access to the database and subschemas are applied when others need to see the same database. If the individual records need to be linked, this connection must be explained and to what extent the connection needs to be made.

**Data manipulation language**

Data manipulation language (DML) is applied to databases to make manipulating the database user friendly. The use of a DML makes it unnecessary to learn programming language in order to make changes to a database. Query languages are created to allow the user to access information within the database. Natural query languages are the easiest to use because English words are applied to the information within the database and are used when asking the database to retrieve information for manipulation. These words can be typed in or spoken into the computer. In query-by-example (QBE), information tables are created that hold defined pieces of information. The user asks the computer to show information based on selecting information from the predefined tables. The database is searched based on the selections and the result can be seen by the user. Structured query language (SQL) is used by programmers who know the logical names of information within a database. The user can instruct the computer to find information based on its logical name.

### Data dictionary

Every item in the database is definable and these individual definitions are held in the database's data dictionary. The word or words used to describe each piece of information--what kind of character or characters, like numbers or letters--and how much memory is used for each piece of information, is in the data dictionary. The dictionary keeps a record of who can manipulate information in the database and when the information is manipulated. All parts of the computer that access the information are defined in the data dictionary. A passive data dictionary just provides a list of all of the information stored in the dictionary. An active data dictionary is linked to applications within the system, so if it is manipulated, so are the applications that are linked to it.

### Data security

Privacy or confidentiality protection of databases is important in the healthcare field because information in the databases is personal and most patients would not want their private information accessed by anyone outside of the healthcare field. Management must protect individual records and the database in its entirety. Passwords are the most common way to limit numerous people from obtaining private information. If a whole database full of patients needs to be analyzed, the patients' personal information can be removed leaving their case information but with no names or personal identifying information attached. Virus protection is necessary because people try to intentionally harm or completely ruin databases and operating systems. Networks and floppy disks are the main avenues through which viruses are passed so software should be installed to protect the system. Data backup and recovery systems ensure that information maintained in the healthcare computer system is saved and can be retrieved for later use. Keeping a record of where the information is stored is important so, if necessary, the information can be accessed and can be investigated in case of unauthorized access.

### Object-oriented databases

At times in the healthcare setting there is a need to not only have access to text, but the ability to attach graphs or other objects to the text. Binary large objects (BLOBs) connect images to text in relational databases, but only the text remains searchable.

Object-oriented databases are a new technology that would make the objects and the text searchable. An object-oriented database management system (OODBMS) provides a fast way to access images and sound information and can understand multiple programming languages. Unfortunately, the database in an OODBMS is not as protected as in a relational database and the numbers of searches allowed are not as advanced. Healthcare industries such as genetics, telemedicine and educational medical facilities have used object-oriented databases to link text with objects and integrate programming languages.

**Hypermedia and distributed databases**

Besides object-oriented databases, there are hypermedia databases which can provide access to objects, video and audio files. Hypermedia databases work in the same way that hypertext databases do. A word or phrase within a sentence (referred to as a node) can be clicked on and will take the user to a link to access the information contained within the node. If a demonstration of a procedure can help a person more accurately understand the procedure, the creator of the document can provide a link to the video using a hypermedia database. The healthcare industry uses hypermedia databases in medical teleconferencing meetings. If storing information on a multitude of computer systems in various locations is necessary, a distributed database can be used. A distributed database allows for space to be added so the database can grow and remain working if one of its contributing databases stops working. Because there are many databases working together, managing the entire database can be complicated. There are many users accessing the distributed databases and the more people with access, the greater chance of a security problem.

In a distributed database, many different locations have separate databases that are all working together. A patient's information may be stored in several databases and a doctor may need to see the patient's entire medical history. Finding and obtaining the information can be difficult because the databases are dispersed. Data warehouses are databases that contain all of the patient's important information in one place so the information can be accessed when necessary. The healthcare industry uses a clinical data repository (CDR) to maintain patient's records; including when they seek healthcare, their financial status with the medical facility, the conclusion of tests performed on the patient and surgical procedures pertaining to the heart. The University of Virginia uses the CDR as a way to research and maintain accurate patient records including death rates and what procedures are the most successful. If a particular piece of data requires specific analysis, a data mart can be created to meet the needs of various departments or users. Data marts can come from information in data warehouses, or if a data mart becomes large enough it can lead to the creation of a data warehouse.

Problems surrounding separate transactional and research platforms, incorrect data entry and the use of various types of computers can arise when creating and using data warehouses. A data warehouse stores information in a main database, but the information contained in the database needs to be used for a variety of purposes. Some people in the industry need to input and access separate pieces of patient information, while researchers need to analyze the database as a whole. The needs of both groups are important and software has been created to make the data warehouse acceptable to both. Because there are many databases being accessed that contribute to the data warehouse, mistakes in entering data are common, which can cause searchable information to be lost. A master patient index (MPI) can be used to identify the patient's records with numbers that all people who access the database use. Different parts of the healthcare organization use different types of computers, which may not communicate with one another. Technology standards such as the Health Level-7 and Systematized Nomenclature of Medical Reference Terminology are used to make sure healthcare organizations use information that can be linked in data warehouses.

**Computer-based medical records**

Every person who has ever seen a doctor for any reason has a unique medical record. The record details what procedures and diagnoses a patient has received and keeps a history of the patient's medical information. A medical record serves as a place for patient history and as a source of information for research and study. Computer-based patient records, or CPR's, have become an important means of maintaining patients' medical records away from keeping paper files and most members of the healthcare industry have created computerized records for the patients' medical history. The process is not complete and most organizations have only some of the information stored in computer files. Cost is a major concern for implementing completely computerized records and some providers doubt that it is necessary. Some argue that only information important to research should be computerized. Progress is being made toward a system of computer-based patient records, but the level of advancement varies greatly among healthcare organizations.

## Order entry and results reporting software

Within a healthcare organization, communication between departments is necessary because all medical treatments are not performed in one office. For example, a pregnant woman needs to have blood drawn from a lab. The doctor must make this request and be able to receive communication from the lab with the conclusion reached by the tests. This communication is achieved through computer software programs called order-entry and results-reporting software. Order-entry software must be easy to understand and easy to use because either a doctor or his administrative staff will be inputting requests into the system. Because there is an abundance of communication that must be entered into the system, it must be fast and efficient. The system allows for typed rather than written instructions, which can help improve communication between doctors and lab technicians or pharmacists who no longer have to read and decipher a doctor's handwriting. This helps improve patient care.

## Information technology systems

The increasing price of medical supplies needed to provide adequate healthcare services are being passed on to the patients and companies who provide healthcare to their employees. The result is that fewer people can afford coverage and an increasing number of employers are discontinuing their healthcare coverage. The widespread use of the internet has provided an avenue for people to research and get information about healthcare issues. Because there is accurate and inaccurate information available online, the healthcare industry should create strategies so patients can get correct information from the internet. Information technology should be used to help reduce or eliminate healthcare-related mistakes. Evidence-based medicine, or EBM, can be provided with the use of the computer. EBM is a collaborative database of conclusions based on patient cases that can be used as a source for healthcare providers. Protecting a patient's personal information has to be a priority in order for healthcare providers to follow guidelines set forth by the Health Insurance Portability and Accountability Act, or HIPAA.

HIPAA, or the Health Insurance Portability and Accountability Act require changes to not only new information technology systems, but require immediate changes to computer security systems. The guidelines set forth by HIPAA require healthcare providers to better protect the private information of individual patients. Clinical information systems are databases with patient diagnoses and information about how each patient's case is being handled by the provider. These systems need to be upgraded and streamlined. The usage of the internet to advertise and recruit employees will continue to grow for healthcare practices. Information technology that can be used wirelessly is in greater demand and wireless technology will continue to be in demand. The internet is currently a great source of patient information and customer relationship management (CRM) systems. CRM systems, that provide information to patients based on their diagnosis and problems are being developed. A well-developed CRM system will provide access to patient's medical information, to the patient and anyone involved in the patient's healthcare management.

The systems theory can be described as the basis for information technology in healthcare. Based on this theory, information technology systems can be analyzed on their total performance and how each performs quantitatively in comparison to others. Systems related to healthcare are divided into 3 groups, which are mechanical systems, human systems, and man-machine systems. Mechanical systems include the systems necessary for a healthcare organization to function mechanically, including the capability of maintaining the physical environments of the organization. A human system applies to a system relating to people, including patients and physicians and their relationships. Man-machine systems are systems that are used to aid a person in the healthcare process. An ultrasound machine which monitors a baby's heartbeat is a man-machine system. Information systems are either human or man-machine systems. If a system does not require a computer to analyze input it is called a manual system.

The 7 concepts that define a system are:

(1) A system is something that has oneness and can be described based on its unique characteristics. A system will be its own entity and elicit a precise description.
(2) A system contains interwoven parts that are numerous and rely on each other for the system to function. A healthcare system will have many levels and each level can be broken down into smaller levels.
(3) A system will change when necessary and resist deterioration when system upgrades are necessary.
(4) A system must be able to react to defined situations and to situations that are not defined. It must be adaptable to human needs.
(5) The system must be able to receive information, process the information and provide a response to the information.
(6) The system has to be able to adjust itself to the response or output it provides, a process that is referred to as feedback.

(7) An open system can be affected by external sources while a closed system is self-contained and cannot be affected by outside sources.

A system must have a built-in component that will identify areas where improvement is necessary. A healthcare system will count the number of services provided and determine to what degree of excellence the services were provided. The system will measure how much support was required to provide the services. Some of the information fed into the system will be predetermined and fit a schedule, while other will be spontaneous, based on needs that develop with patient care. A management control will measure these standards against standards of management created to ensure quality of care was upheld. If the established standards are not met, the system control will suggest changes to improve the process. The system standards are typically created collaboratively by management and employees who work in the field. The standards are dynamic and must be monitored and changed continuously to maintain an up-to-date and successful environment. The Joint Commission on Accreditation of Healthcare Organizations creates standards that are input into healthcare systems to ensure compliance.

Information systems are designed to help a healthcare organization (HCO) provide quality care. The computer systems are designed to help healthcare providers by providing information which can direct the user's actions or let the user know when a potential mistake in input has occurred. The systems provide healthcare providers a source of information including the HCO's protocols and other necessary job-related information. The information system is also designed to track data so management can see areas for improvement and ensure expected results are met. The computer systems should be able to process and store information and should be able to provide illness-specific information when requested. Because both requirements are necessary, the healthcare field is requiring the computer to think through diagnoses and treatments and serve administrative functions. Information systems are being developed that can support both functions.

## Information system strategies

The four reasons why a healthcare organization should develop strategies regarding the use of information technology include the following: to ensure the information technology is best used to meet an organization's standards, to make sure the computer systems are being used at their optimum value, to manipulate the computer systems technologically to meet the unique goals of the organization, and to determine how much money will be spent on the computer systems. Information technology has always been used to perform functions helping a healthcare organization with normal activities like scheduling appointments. Healthcare managers can use information systems to meet goals such as bringing in more patients or monitoring patient wait times. Because every organization's goals are tailored for their specific organization, the technology needed will vary and should be evaluated to make sure it includes the right systems for the organization. Determining the type of network an organization needs and understanding how to use the network most effectively should be part of the organization's plan.

An information system is so important to a healthcare organization that many levels of experts should be consulted before a decision is made as to what type of system the organization will use. The highest of senior management should have oversight and he or she should develop a workgroup, called a steering committee, to help research and decide on an appropriate selection. The steering committee may be part of healthcare management and should include people from diverse departments who will be able to articulate the capabilities each will require of an information system. The members of the committee should know best what is needed to make their department successful in the overall goals of the organization. The finer details should be left for subcommittees who should have specifically designated tasks, like defining how the network can actually function, and the steps needed for implementation. If necessary, people who are knowledgeable and work in the information technology field outside of the healthcare organization should be brought in to give advice to the committees. Their specialized training in computers and healthcare should be used when considering the choice and implementation of a system.

Part of the planning process for the use of an information technology system should include the format information will take when entered into the computer system. A data dictionary can be created which gives examples of and defines the format of data; when a user needs to enter information, the dictionary can be consulted. Information is exchanged between the departments of an organization and between medically-related businesses outside of the organization. This creates the need for use of the same type of data language, providing the systems with the ability to exchange information. Because this is an important issue for the healthcare industry as a whole, groups like The American National Standards Institute and the Health Industry Bar Code Supplier Labeling Standard have been formed to create common data formats. The recommendations made by these groups are not required for implementation, but can help with data congruency. The Health Insurance Portability and Accountability Act (HIPAA) has made some information formats standard.

Once an area of need is discovered concerning information technology within a healthcare organization, a team of specific people within the organization should be formed to work together in addressing the problem--a process called project organization. A top executive should maintain oversight over each member of the team and the overall project. An expert from the information technology department should have oversight and manage the people working on the project. Experts from every business unit who will be affected by the use of a new system should have input on the project including doctors, department leaders, and information technology personnel. A person who can communicate the expert's resolutions with the top executive overseeing the project should be available. Sometimes a healthcare organization does not have the manpower to oversee a project on their own and must hire an outside company to perform the task. The structure of people involved in the project should remain consistent whether completed within the organization or outside of the organization.

**Information system development**

Information technology applications are complex and evolve over time. The first step in the development of an information system requires managers to figure out all the information they can about the system the organization is using--a process called systems analysis. It is difficult to improve a system without knowing its current capabilities and shortfalls. A wish- list of the performance functions of the new system should be created within this step. The analysis of different types of new systems and the current system and their individual pros and cons should be created. All of the information should be combined and analyzed to determine the best course of action for the organization. This should be presented in writing to the decision-making executives. The executives should read over the information and give their authorization in writing so the next step of the process can begin.

As the system is evaluated in the first step of the computer life cycle process, information must be gathered and put into an understandable format for evaluation. To discover the strengths and weaknesses of the system currently being used, a main source of information can be the people using the system on a daily basis. Time should be spent talking to the employees to determine the issues they face and the things they like about the computer system. How the work unit functions should be determined through gathering information from the workforce because the processes used must be incorporated into a new computer system. Once the information is gathered, it must be compiled so management can understand what is being presented. A step-by-step picture called a flowchart of the current system can show where improvement is needed. Written reports and visual displays can help management clearly understand the results.

Management can use the information they have gathered to decide what kind of system they will need--whether it be a custom-designed system or one that already exists--in the second step of the life cycle development process. Evaluating price is a major factor in this step. A package that is complete and ready for use may not function exactly the way an organization needs it to and must be altered in some ways. Any alterations cost money in both manpower and technology. The price may seem less than a custom-designed program until the costs of alterations are added in. Making a system that is custom-designed by either people employed within an organization or a company outside of the organization may be a better option. Huge organizations with many departments and employees will have a difficult time finding a preexisting system that meets all of the needs of their organization.

The third step of the process is to prepare the organization by determining what technology is needed for the new computer system--a process called system design. Whether the organization uses a program that is already developed or one that is custom designed, the system requirements or specifications must be communicated for the system to work. If technicians within the organization are going to create the system, certain areas should be considered. What is needed from the system, how the system should give and receive information (known as output and input), and storage of the information within databases should all be determined. Determining how all system parts will communicate with each other effectively is another part of system design. Being able to show management their money is well spent and gaining their written approval are the last steps of the process of creating a system within an organization. If hiring a company outside of the organization to create the system, a report specifying needs and wants should be created and provided to the hired company.

The fourth step of the process requires gathering everything that will be needed to create the system, including software and hardware or purchasing the system from an outside source. If buying a previously designed system, each component should be investigated for price comparison and system capabilities. People who have applied the various systems to their organizations should be questioned as to how adaptable the system was to their organization and any problems they have experienced. The Internet is another great source of information and many opinions and technical information can be found by searching different Internet sources.

Those studying the different systems should determine if the company providing the system will help integrate the system within the organization and what resources they have to help if something goes wrong with the system. Software will be needed to make the system run and the software will have different prices attached to it that must be considered.

Once a system has been chosen and designed, the system must be put into use, which is the fifth step in the developmental process--called system implementation. This step involves having someone available to show new users how to manipulate and work with the computer system. The system's performance should be evaluated, by having the users perform normal processes to ensure the system is working effectively. Elements of the system, such as hardware and software, should be assessed for efficiency while being used. Another area that should be assessed is the monetary price of running the system; this cost should be compared to the organization's expectations. During the fifth step, information needed from the old system should be input into the new system. The new database should be created and management should decide what to do with the old computer databases. The supplies needed for the system should be purchased and set up.

The sixth step requires the oversight of the implemented system so potential problems can be solved and maintenance can be performed to avoid potential future problems. Typically this requires hiring system experts to address problems when they arise; system problems, especially during implementation, are common problems. These experts should be available to manipulate the system to meet the needs of the organization after implementation. It is important for communication to occur between those people creating the system and those who maintain it. If a group within the organization creates a system, they should create training material for the system, or train the people maintaining it. If an outside organization creates the system, they should communicate how to maintain the system. A strategy should be created and communicated in case the system fails--called a backup plan. The personnel and information technology employees must be trained on what to do in case the system fails to work for any reason.

The seventh step requires management to determine if the system could be made better to match the needs of the healthcare agency. New policies, procedures and management vision can all affect the needs required of the system. The theory that nothing is ever perfect and can be consistently made better is referred to as total quality management (TQM). TQM should be applied while judging the system. It is important to determine if the system is working as expected and providing for the needs of every department it was created for. The ease with which employees can use the system and their happiness with it should be considered. The price of the system versus how it has bettered the organization is another area for analysis. Finally, how many problems occur with the system should be determined and assessed against expectations.

## Bargaining and contracts

During the selection process in the fourth stage of the system-development life cycle, many companies are being evaluated for selection by the healthcare organization. Typically, a couple of companies lead the pack in what they have to offer. While the healthcare company bargains for who can give them the best deal, it is acceptable to let one company know what the other is offering and let the companies fight for the healthcare organization's business. All paperwork committing the healthcare organization to a company should be screened by lawyers employed by the healthcare organization to assure the organization is protected. Consequences for the outside technology company not meeting the agreed-upon bid should be detailed in a legal document. When the system will be available, proof that it works, when financial obligations will be met, are all areas that should be covered in the legal agreement. Other areas, such as how long the outside company will support the system, possession of software title, and the length of the contract, should also be addressed.

## Information system management

The healthcare industry places huge demands on information technology, because computer systems are used in a variety of departments and locations--both alongside the patient at a facility and away from a facility--either with a patient at an outside location or in a business meeting held away from the office. Management has to develop approaches in a meaningful and direct way to manage and oversee information systems currently in use and those needed for future use. It is imperative for the healthcare organization's management to carefully consider how much money will be spent on information systems and where in the organization will benefit from its use. Another area management must consider is how to integrate different types of systems, thus creating congruency within healthcare systems. Not doing this wastes time and money because input can be duplicated and human resources are required to input potentially unnecessary information.

## Application service providers

Companies who cannot afford to buy a system or make one themselves may need to pay an outside company who owns the required system applications to use their technology. These companies are called application service providers (ASPs) and the companies offer access to their information technology via the Internet. The systems are ready to use but cannot typically be modified for the needs of a specific organization. The fee to use the service is negotiated and set so the organization will know how much it is paying every month rather than guessing at how much maintaining an owned system will cost. The use of an outside company for the information technology needs of a healthcare organization means that the outside company will have access to private organizational and patient information, so the integrity of the company must be researched and evaluated before it is chosen.

## Laboratory automation and laboratory information systems

Laboratory automation is the process by which computers send and receive data from laboratory instruments. The tools used in a laboratory must automatically communicate their results to a computer which can decipher the results and create a report for the lab technician to analyze. The use of software programs rather than hardware equipment in laboratory automation is cheaper and is becoming more widely used. Clinical labs use laboratory automation while other types of labs use laboratory information systems to keep track of and maintain test results. Laboratory information systems have the capability of analysis, which saves on human resources needed to perform the same function. How and when lab tests are performed is detailed in laboratory information systems. If a record of tests completed on a patient is required, the system will provide the information. The results can be printed out and shared among various departments saving time and money.

## Pharmacy information systems

Because pharmacists and pharmacy technicians are responsible for controlled substances, the organization of medicine within the pharmacy is very important. Files must be maintained to ensure the right amount of medicine is given to patients and so the information can be tracked. Smaller pharmacies that are not part of large chains can use stand-alone pharmacy computer systems that maintain records for drugs within the pharmacy. The computer system only has to record information of drugs distributed from one location. Some pharmacies are connected to hospitals or other healthcare providers, so a computer system must be used that is part of a larger computer application. Maintaining records is especially important when it comes to drugs because mistakes are common. Some drugs cannot be taken with other drugs; also, the correct dosage must be dispensed by the pharmacist. There are many types of pharmacy information systems available and healthcare providers should choose programs with built-in defenses against common prescription mistakes.

### Medical imaging and radiology information systems

Through the use of medical imaging systems and radiology information systems, doctors have the ability to view images more extensively and the continued development of the products is very important to the healthcare industry. Pictures can be taken and manipulated with medical imaging systems. Patient exams, including when they will occur and the outcome of the exam, are produced by radiology information systems. Radiology information systems can compile information for management needs. The computer has the ability to help doctors in the field of radiology by giving the doctors several possibilities when determining the best way to handle a patient's problems. The doctor can zoom into pictures and input different treatment plans to determine the best way to handle a case. Picture archiving and communication systems (PACS) are present in radiology departments because they store radiology pictures and can be quickly accessed by users. Teleradiology equipment allows the physician to move pictures from one location to another or view the pictures away from the radiology office.

### Ambulatory care information systems

There is a demand for computer systems that support offices with one doctor and larger offices that have merged several doctors in a single location. Ambulatory care information systems are important because information can be entered from a remote location. Smaller offices need computers to perform basic functions like maintaining appointments, billing and allowing users to type reports and keep patient medical information. Large practices see a large number of patients and need patient information to be stored and organized electronically. The computer systems each doctor's staff uses must be compatible with those of other doctors in the practice so the billing information and patient records can be shared throughout the office. Hospitals are being connected with the computer systems of large practices so the office can prepare patients for admittance to the hospital directly from the doctor's office. This provides a convenience to the patients and the doctor offices enjoy providing the service to their patients.

**Nursing information systems**

Nursing information systems help nurses determine the best patient care, oversee critical patients, and oversee groups of nurses. Nurses can input a patient's symptoms into a protocol-based computer system and the computer will output different treatments that may help the patient. The patient's record can be maintained through the computer and the system can track a patient's care electronically rather than manually. Nurses must be educated on the use of the system in order for it to be most effective. Point-of-care computer systems that can be used wherever the patient is seen by the nurse provide many benefits. A nurse has the ability to complete his or her record keeping while with the patient rather than writing notes and inputting the information later leading to fewer errors in the transfer of information. Laptops and other portable computers can be used by nurses to input medical information.

**Clinical decision-support systems**

Discovering the cause of a patient's symptoms and the best way to relieve the patient's symptoms can be investigated by doctors through the use of clinical decision-support systems (CDSS). Passive CDSS computer systems accept medical information, but cannot make changes or produce outcomes based on the information. Passive CDSS systems organize the information in a functional and orderly fashion so the doctor can easily analyze the patient's information. Rather than having to flip through paper charts that have the patient's medical history and current problems, the CDSS provides the information in a central location. In an active CDSS, the computer has the ability to help the doctor with research and patient evaluation. Known medical information is stored in the active CDSS so the computer can analyze patient's problems and apply known medical treatments to give the doctor some suggestions for how best to treat the patient.

Active CDSS systems include expert systems, probabilistic algorithm systems and clinical reminder and alert systems. Expert systems consist of a general knowledge base, patient-specific information and a rule-based inference engine. Each area of medicine has people with a high degree of knowledge about their related field of medicine. Their knowledge is included in the general knowledge base of the expert system. Patient-specific information is compared to the general knowledge base.

The rule-based inference engine applies all known information and gives the doctor suggestions for care. Statistical probabilities based on previous case outcomes rather than expert knowledge is produced by the probabilistic algorithms part of the expert system. Expert systems include clinical reminders to alert the care provider of possible problems with treatments or medical problems that can arise as a result of a treatment plan.

### Computer-assisted medical instrumentation

Many instruments for use in medical offices and hospitals are computer-assisted. Computer-assisted medical instrumentation means that the equipment can be connected to and communicate with a computer. Patients are connected directly to machines in many settings so the computer can keep track of heart monitoring, blood pressure, respiratory rates and other related patient measurements. The information is placed in computer memory so the computer can track and compile data for the user to request. Software is available that can modify or produce results based on the user's request. The data received by the equipment can be sent to a main terminal or any location that is linked to the system, including a patient's computerized chart if available. Anesthesiologists use decision-support systems to monitor the amount of medication a patient is receiving during a procedure. Devices used for heart and lung procedures are connected to computer systems to record the progress of treatment during and after a procedure.

### Telemedicine and teleradiology

Some patients do not have access to a medical facility either because they are too sick or live too far away from a physician's office. Medical caregivers can travel to these patients and administer healthcare with the use of remote computer systems which is a process called telemedicine. The patient's information can be transmitted using wireless technology. Pictures can be taken remotely and transferred to experts in the radiology fields; this process is known as teleradiology. The use of telemedicine is more cost effective than creating a medical center that every person in every location has access to and specialists can be consulted through the use of the technology. The University of California Davis Medical Center is using telemedicine to track heart patients in remote locations, allowing the patients to live at home rather than in a hospital setting. Some health insurance companies are still hesitant in reimbursing patients for telemedicine and it is sometimes difficult to keep the patient's medical information secure when being accessed remotely.

### Long-term care and home healthcare information systems

Long-term care information systems are being used in facilities like nursing homes and assisted living homes. Because the patients of long-term care facilities require constant monitoring, the systems have been improved to update the patient's records quickly so the patient's record is constantly maintained with current information. The future of long-term care information systems should include the ability for the system to communicate with outside medical facilities so a patient's information can be quickly sent to an emergency room or other medical center if necessary. Information systems are being used for home healthcare situations so a healthcare provider can use a portable device to enter a patient's information at the site of service, which saves time and reduces errors. Computer systems are used to research the causes of diseases and maintain records of treatments and cases so students can study real life situations. A computer can compile and compare data faster and more accurately than humans, making research capabilities better than ever before. MEDLINE is a database where physicians can share experiences and data collection for the purpose of research by fellow medical colleagues and students.

### Financial information systems

Financial information systems are important to the healthcare industry because the industry is subject to government oversight and there are many providers offering the same type of services, which creates a competitive environment. Financial information systems have the ability to track costs and produce reports so management can make sound financial decisions for their organization. Daily activity regarding finances is submitted into the computer's transaction-processing systems, one part of the financial information system. Data from external sources, including government and market data, is another part of the financial information system. Strategic organization plans that are unique to the financial mission of each healthcare location are the third part of the financial information system. All parts of the financial information system work together so complete oversight of the organization's finances is achieved. For a financial information system to be successful, the input data must be accurate and complete. The accounting program an organization uses must be of high quality. Payment programs vary between monthly payments and payment by treatment, so the system must be flexible and have the ability to consider all types of payment options.

## Human resources information systems

A good human resources information system (HRIS) is vital to the healthcare industry because it is largely a service industry and there are many people working for pay and benefits. Each person working for the industry has a file stored in a database that must be accessed continuously which is part of the HRIS. The employees' identifying information and work history are stored within these files. The number of people working in the organization, the quality of their work, training and education, and the cost of human resources and payment for their services must all be tracked with the HRIS. The information contained in the HRIS is sensitive and confidentiality must be maintained through the use of hardware and software. Management should be able to use the HRIS system to assess how the human resources are functioning including the rate at which they are leaving the company or getting terminated and the level of happiness they have with their jobs.

## Executive information system

The main leaders of an organization have to make sure every department is functioning properly and that the overall output of their organization is satisfactory to the owners of the organization. An executive information system (EIS) is designed to monitor how all of the areas within an organization are functioning and provides upper management a way to retrieve the data as a whole or in smaller pieces to be analyzed. The data warehouse must be managed so it will contain the data needed for the reports. Executives will not access an EIS unless they can easily use the program and have the ability to manipulate the data as they desire. The EIS has to be able to give the leaders the reports they need, so communication between leadership and those creating the DSS is especially important. Training is vital so the benefits of using the EIS system--rather than traditional and known tools used by management--are taught to employees.

## Computerized resource utilization and scheduling systems

To keep costs minimized all resources must be used accurately and efficiently. Managers have to make a profit while explaining their resource management to health insurance providers and government agencies monitoring their use of resources. Scheduling systems are important because part of making a profit requires having healthcare providers with time to perform procedures and visit patients. Both resource utilization and scheduling systems have been computerized so oversight of the two essential areas is more efficient. To ensure resources such as bed space and room space are available and used efficiently, advance bed booking and pre-admission systems are used. In order for Medicare to pay for services, the services must be pre-approved and advanced booking allows the healthcare organization time to make sure the services are covered. The future of computerized resource utilization and scheduling systems involve a wider use by all departments within an organization. The systems will perform functions currently performed by people, like making sure a patient is insured and the oversight of human resource needs.

Physicians' offices that are linked to hospital computer systems can input admissions information before the admission date, allowing hospitals to know how many beds will be used on a given day. Not only will scheduling systems help determine bed availability, but they can also help the organization know how many caregivers are needed to provide service. If a specific area is low in patients, some employees who work flexible schedules will not be required to come to work, which saves the facility in the cost of manpower. Operating rooms are a specific area of a hospital that must be scheduled for use and computer scheduling systems can provide this service. This helps reduce the problem of equipment being needed in more than one room--because the rooms are scheduled and the schedule can be easily accessed in the system. Some organizations operate at many clinics and physicians rotate around the clinics providing services. This requires a need for outpatient clinic appointment and scheduling systems that can keep track of each doctor's schedule and location among the clinics.

## Materials management systems

Materials management systems are computer programs that help management oversee the usage and payment of medical supplies. A budget is established by the organization and input into the computer system. When medical equipment is needed, it is requested through the system and the system can determine if funds are available for the purchase. If there is not enough money to make the purchase, management will be notified by the system so they can approve or deny the order. The computer can produce purchase requests and monitor when the supplies are received based on matching materials to what has been requested and purchased. The Internet has provided an avenue for the healthcare organization's computer system to communicate requests directly to vendors of medical supplies. Barcodes are the common device used to track materials within the computer system because they are easily scanned, sending the information into the computer. Menu-planning systems can help oversee food menus and the nutritional needs of patients.

## Facilities and project management systems

Most healthcare services are provided from a physical location and computerized facilities and project management systems are designed to oversee various aspects of the location. One type of system controls preventative maintenance ensuring that equipment is consistently working properly and necessary maintenance is completed. When equipment is maintained there are fewer problems, which can save the organization money in parts, labor, and safety problems. Another type of system control manages and reports energy usage, helping management oversee how energy costs can be reduced to save money. As buildings deteriorate, they must be updated and project management system controls help with the construction in healthcare buildings. Program Evaluation and Review Technique (PERT) is an established program which tracks the progress and cost of details regarding a construction project. The program can set deadlines based on completion goals and make adjustments based on actual progress.

## Office automation systems and groupware

Documentation is a huge part of the healthcare field because patient and employee files must be kept within an office. Before office automation, paper files were kept on each patient and employee and the files had to be organized and maintained in a way that people could retrieve and re-file the paper documents. Management of the documents took time and money to pay salaries for the employees responsible for the job. Office automation can be used to connect departments and maintain records for multiple departments within an organization through the use of e-mail and electronic scheduling programs. Groupware can be defined as hardware and software that is designed to work together to join departments, especially by communication. Groupware is used in the healthcare industry to share information between departments and managers.

## Managed care

When a group of doctors or practices provide medical care to a set of defined people, the doctors are said to be involved in managed care. Health maintenance organizations (HMOs) are physicians that see patients within a specific insurance plan for a prearranged price set between the insurance company and HMO. A preferred provider organization (PPO) is a physician who provides medical services for a lower cost to a predefined group of people. If a person under a PPO insurance plan sees a doctor within the PPO network the medical services will be charged by the PPO at a lower rate. Exclusive provider arrangements (EPAs) are developed when a company pays a specific physician to provide medical services to all of their employees without the use of an insurance company. Managed care plans are offered at various prices and coverage options so management must research and find the best type of coverage for their organization.

It is imperative that computer systems in a managed healthcare setting provide purchasers, consumers, providers and managed care organizations with answers to questions each group has. Purchasers, or people buying coverage for a group of people, including federal and state governments who buy insurance coverage for Medicare and Medicaid members, need to know several pieces of information. The type of coverage provided, the price of the healthcare, how good the insurance is, and who uses the plan, are all areas that purchasers need to know about. Consumers include employees who may have a choice in coverage providers and they need to know answers to questions in the same areas the purchasers investigate, as well as what plan is the most accessible and easiest to use. Providers and managed care organizations work together and need to know unique information about the managed care programs. Providers need to know their profit margins, how many patients are being seen per membership in a managed care organization and how they will be paid. Managed care organizations need to know how best to sell their services, how much they should charge, and how many people, and who, are using their plans. All of the data can be part of a managed care information system.

**Quality of care**

Employers and employees care greatly about how good their health insurance coverage is. Employers who are purchasing healthcare plans want to provide the best possible care for the employees who work for them and are also paying a portion of insurance premiums. Accreditation agencies have been developed to investigate and report on HMO's service. The National Committee on Quality Assurance (NCQA) is an accreditation agency that oversees the overall quality of care through measuring many different aspects of HMO's. The measurements are recorded on the agencies' Health Plan Employer Data and Information Set. Computerized quality of care programs are being developed to track patient's care to determine how good or bad it is. Computerized claims processing helps the processing of billing and payment tracking to become a more streamlined and efficient process. The provider using electronic claims processing can quickly see if a patient is covered for a procedure by his or her insurance company. Claims made to health insurance companies have to be electronically submitted per the Health Insurance Portability and Accountability Act (HIPAA).

### Integrated delivery systems

Integrated delivery systems (IDSs) consist of different types of physicians and hospitals joining together to provide a variety of healthcare to certain established groups of people. Communication between the members of an IDS is key and computer information systems must be created that are compatible with many different types of already established computer systems. Before the creation of the IDS group, the offices were separate entities with their own unique systems and must be brought together into one main computer system after they merge. Patient records must be viewed by multiple providers involved in the IDS. The computer network has to support a specific number of locations, have the ability to store information, allow for real-time communication, and provide a protected environment for the users. An alternative to the expensive venture of changing all computer systems into a single system is using software like an enterprise index and enterprise scheduling system.

### E-business applications

E-health is used to describe how the Internet has been increasingly used in the healthcare field in many areas to make overall healthcare better. E-business applications include e-procurement, electronic claims processing and consumer e-business. E-business applications provide communication between providers of medical care and people who do business with medical providers outside of providing patient care. E-procurement occurs when a medical provider buys equipment and merchandise over the Internet needed for their practice to function. Electronic claims processing occurs when the healthcare provider and insurance provider communicate over the Internet about patient coverage and billing. Consumer e-business involves the use of the Internet to buy healthcare-related items without a healthcare provider being involved in the transaction. Medication that normally requires a prescription and insurance can be bought over the Internet.

### Marketing and consumer information applications

Healthcare providers use the Internet to discuss their practices and discuss healthcare trends with potential and current customers through the use of marketing and consumer information applications. Marketing a doctor's office and the services they provide is common through the use of websites on the Internet. The information contained on the website can be made searchable and the website can be advertised in traditional marketing like a Yellow Pages ad. Consumers can find out the doctor's experience and education and what procedures the doctor can perform. Some websites offer general health information and articles for those interested and many will list the insurances the practice accepts. Consumer health information is provided via the Internet by the government and private companies. Healthfinder.gov is a huge database created buy the U.S. Department of Health and Human Services that contains information on a variety of health related services.

**Organizational management and communications applications**

Organizational management and communications applications are used within company Intranets and their uses include distributing organizational information, education and training, employee recruiting, and administrative operations. Departmental communication is important to a healthcare industry. The industry is constantly developing new strategies and implementing new rules that must be communicated to the staff so they can be followed. The Intranet is commonly used to communicate new information to the employees, saving the organization money from buying paper and ink to print every new piece of information. Documents, like healthcare paperwork and IRS forms can be accessed on the Intranet so they are only printed when needed. Education and training materials and video programs can be delivered through the Intranet so a trainer can deliver the information once and it can be communicated whenever necessary. Human resources generally post job openings within the organization that internal employees can access. Administrative operations like word processing and financial reports can be conducted through the computer.

**Decision-support system**

Decision support can be defined as a way to use specific information to help a person determine the best course of action in handling any issues that arise. The key to decision support is using known information and evaluating the information to make a decision rather than using experience or feelings. Decision support can be done manually or through the use of a computer application that can process information. Gathering and analyzing data manually can be time consuming and difficult for management who do not have the human resources available to help in the process. There are many steps involved in analyzing different possibilities when coming to a decision. Using a specifically designed program referred to as a decision-support system that can get data, combine and decipher the data, come to a decision, apply various pros and cons to the decision and make sound recommendations can save time and money. Decision-support systems can help management come to better decisions more quickly.

A decision-support system (DSS) contains the following elements: user interface, model manager, model library, database, database-management system and a report writer. Data is input into the DSS through the user interface. Because management typically inputs the data, the user interface must be user friendly. A model manager is the part of the DSS that accesses information that has been created to evaluate a problem. The model library contains the various models used to analyze a problem including the use of math, visual displays, financial and models that determine possible outcomes if a decision is applied. The DSS gets information from a database which is usually a relational database. The database-management system oversees and guides the communication between the user and the database. The outcomes of using the DSS are provided to the user through the report writer.

Alter defined several areas where the use of a DSS is applicable. If the DSS system is just needed to get a specific piece of information, a DSS that can search a database is needed. If an ad hoc study or a study of a specifically defined piece of information is required of a DSS system, any system that performs mathematical analysis can be used. If information needs to be compiled into a single output, an executive information system can be used. A DSS has to be able to perform "what-if" analysis if a manager needs to see different outcomes based on input scenarios. In order to have a DSS system that gives recommendations to the user, it must be a system that can process information providing the best possible outcomes. Some systems can actually analyze data and produce an outcome that is not just a recommendation but a conclusion that can be relied upon. These applications need a DSS system that is capable of intelligent retrieval.

A decision-support system (DSS) contains facts about many different categories of information. These facts that are entered into the computer must be determined by management and must cover healthcare clients, collective healthcare information, data that changes over time and information that can be measured against other similar data. A DSS can be used in a healthcare organization when management is trying to determine their best tactical plan for conducting business in the future, also known as a strategic plan. The information needed to develop future approaches includes constant evaluation of other providers offering the same services. Physicians must monitor how much others charge for the same medical care and what makes their services unique when evaluated against others offering the same service.

Interaction between healthcare providers and patients is constantly being recorded through the use of transaction processing systems within the healthcare organization. These systems keep important patient data needed for a DSS system. The amount of people seen and for what purpose can be retrieved for later analysis from the systems. Information that is not kept by transaction processing systems must still be obtained for a DSS system to be complete. This data is typically subjective and surveys must be conducted to get the information. The information must be input into a computer so the DSS system can retrieve it and analyze it. In order for the DSS system to compare data and analyze information based on a community or group of people, information must be entered from origins outside of the office. If information is needed about other healthcare providers, a healthcare organization can chose to research other providers on its own or buy the already collected information from an outside source selling it. Purchasing already collected information is easier, but costs more money and may not include specific information needed for comparison.

In order for a DSS system to be used within a healthcare organization, the organization must buy it and begin using it. A DSS system can be purchased from a supplier that has been designed for immediate use so the healthcare organization can rely on the system to create reports based on built in information. These systems are easy to use but the output is generic. Another type of DSS system can be manipulated by the healthcare organization to provide reports that are unique to whatever problem the organization wants solved. These systems must be altered for use but can give a better-suited report that is unique to the organization. Once chosen, the DSS system must have information to pull from in order to function. A database must be created with information and the database must be able to communicate with the DSS system. Human resources are required to create and oversee the database and ensure the database and DSS are functioning correctly. The organization must then determine how and for what purpose they will use the DSS and begin training employees on how to use the DSS.

**Resource use**

Insurance companies and individuals typically pay healthcare providers based on a set rate charged for each service provided. Insurance companies generally negotiate in advance how much they will pay for each procedure. A DSS system needs data relating to how best each provider should spend his or her money on resources to help the providers save money when buying necessities for their practice. Resources have to be used by the physicians effectively so the best output can be produced while using the least amount of resources. The DSS system can be used to measure the results of how resources are being used, a process known as benchmarking. A healthcare manager who wants to evaluate how his or her practice is functioning in comparison to other practices will use process benchmarking. To make this evaluation, the DSS system needs information such as the actual price the providers are paying for resources and the service level obtained by other providers. The information needed by the DSS system for comparison is often difficult to obtain as healthcare providers measure similar business processes differently.

Both human and non-human resources have to be managed and used effectively by management; a DSS system can help management develop a strategy to best use both resources. By tracking patient volumes, the system can recommend to a manager how many people should be working and at what location at any given time. If more people are needed to provide optimal coverage, the system can recognize the need. A DSS system should have information on how much the healthcare organization is spending on materials and who they are buying the materials from. With that information, the system can make recommendations on the best places and processes available. A DSS system can track how often machines break down and the cause and solution to those problems to determine the best course of action to avoid future problems. A system named CLASSICA has been developed for nurses to oversee and manage resources specific to their job duties.

**Patient care results**

DSS systems are needed to evaluate the outcomes or end results of patient care and how effectively that care has been delivered. There are several different categories of people who want to know these outcomes and each group has a different reason for wanting to know. Healthcare management has to take into account the concerns of each group, including those spending money on the provider's services, those studying the healthcare field, those bridging communication between the physician and patient, the physicians providing the service, and those people receiving the medical attention. The people spending money on the services want to know how much they have to spend and who will perform the service at the best price. Those studying the healthcare field want to know how the providers are affecting the community with their services. The managed care officials want to know which doctors provide the best care at the least amount of cost. The physicians want to make sure they are doing a good job and patients want to know they are getting excellent service. ORYX is a program that evaluates the end results of patient care and is used by the Joint Commission on Accreditation of Healthcare Organizations (JCAHO).

**Finances and advertising**

The use of DSS systems have helped in numerous areas for a variety of businesses. The oversight and analysis of finances in a California-based business selling insurance uses a specifically created DSS system to analyze how best to oversee all finances related to fixed incomes. A healthcare office in Cleveland, Ohio, that provides long-term care for patients needing daily help from a healthcare provider to get better, used a DSS system to determine how a new fee retrieval system would affect their profits. In order to create an effective advertising plan, a company must know who its customers are. Geographic Information Systems (GISs) can be accessed to get information on the people who a business is interested in advertising to. A managed care company in New York used a GIS system to locate which physicians worked in close proximity to people the company was providing healthcare coverage to.

A main source of data required for a DSS system is advertising information. The information needed for the DSS system depends on the medical provider's advertising goals and strategies. Some providers need new business and are considered prospectors because they will search out business instead of waiting for customers to find them. Some providers choose to market by leaning on their performance; this group is known as defenders. Another group of providers, called analyzers, advertise based on what is happening in the marketplace. If a particular service is in high demand, the analyzers will advertise that service. The last group is known as reactors and these providers wait for situations to arise before reacting to them. Reactors do not make hasty advertising decisions but instead use marketing as an afterthought and only when absolutely necessary. Information from both the past and present, including statistics on the people within the market area, is needed for a DSS to cover all of the different groups of medical providers.

**Maximizing profits**

Providing the best services while spending the least amount of money is important in any industry. The healthcare industry must determine ways to maximize profits and one area the industry focuses on is operating efficiently. DSS systems with access to the right information can help oversee and maximize operations. A Jacksonville, Florida, Mayo Clinic relies on a system to oversee and manage the use of their surgical facilities. The information communicated to the system has to be detailed and cover the surgery process from start to finish. Profits are important, but quality must not suffer; if quality suffers, less people will use the services, thus reducing profits. DSS systems are being increasingly used to measure if service is provided in the best possible manner.

**Expert systems**

Expert systems are a type of DSS system that can have authority over and make decisions about areas needing support in the healthcare field. The expert system has several parts including a section with known information, a section that holds information called a database and a section that applies rules to determine possible outcomes. The expert system has an area where information can be input, called a user interface, and a workspace where data is kept. All of the areas work together and communicate with each other in a system. An expert system is meant to be used to solve problems in lieu of human involvement. Expert systems are used in the healthcare industry in a variety of ways, including alerting the organization of out-of-the-ordinary uses of insurance. If, for example, a person lives in Arizona and consistently sees the same set of doctors and the person's insurance cards begin to be used in Florida, an expert system can identify the problem and alert the necessary parties.

**Request for information**

A request for information (RFI) is a verbal or written communication to an information system technology provider used to determine what the company has to offer. The RFI occurs during the fourth step of the development life cycle. If the system needed is not complex, less information is needed for the healthcare organization to choose the best company and the RFI process is referred to as informal. Basic information is shared with the outside company, telling them what the healthcare organization needs from the system. The information technology providers can then tell the healthcare organization if they have the requested technology and, if so, they can provide the healthcare organization with specific price and performance-related information. The information received from the outside companies will be used to compare the products and prices.

## Request for proposal

A request for proposal (RFP) is a written request for information from information technology providers and is used when a complex information technology system is being acquired. RFPs occur during the fourth stage of the development life cycle. The healthcare organization must provide the outside technology provider with information about what it needs from the system--which can be very detailed, or broadly defined. The fewer details provided the more creativity the outside companies can have when creating their suggested course of action. The function of the system, how the company providing the system will be chosen, and overall expectations of the company providing the system should be in the RFPs. How the returned proposals will be evaluated by the healthcare organization should be decided on before the RFPs are sent out. The outside companies should be advised on when they are expected to have their bids ready.

## Secured data

Because computers in the healthcare industry contain personal and private information, they must be guarded through the use of information technology. The computer systems that hold private information are called clinical systems. The computerization of medical records with specific data on people using healthcare services has led to the need for increased security measures. Because certain illnesses are highly contagious and can put many people in danger, these diseases must be monitored through the use of public health information systems. The specific people must still be concealed to avoid derogatory treatment based on their medical condition. To determine trends in the medical field so they can be studied for causes of sicknesses, medical research information systems are used and once again specific individuals' information must be withheld.

## Regulation of privacy

Government control has been used to monitor privacy protection in the healthcare industry. The Health Insurance Portability and Accountability Acct (HIPAA) was passed by the government to control the healthcare industry. A major problem with passing legislation is that, although personal information needs to be protected, laws are passed that state that the information can be shared if there is a threat to a large population of people. For example, a child with AIDS should not have to share that information unless they are placed in a situation like daycare where the illness can potentially be passed on. Legislation may require the child's personal information to be shared in a daycare situation, which essentially fails to protect his or her privacy rights. Non-governmental organizations have tried to set industry standards to be followed by healthcare providers which are meant to safeguard people from having to share their private medical data.

**HIPAA**

Before the Health Insurance Portability and Accountability Act (HIPAA) was enacted, a person could be refused health insurance coverage based on a diagnosed medical problem. The refusal would occur if the person wanted to move from one company to another. HIPAA determined the practice to be unfair and stopped insurance providers from denying medical coverage. Because the personal medical information of patients is contained in computer files, HIPAA regulated the standard of protection required for patient information. Mandating the concealment of medical history will reduce the attempt of insurance companies to discriminate based on the information. Streamlining HIPAA processes across many different healthcare organizations requires HIPAA to define how each organization should comply. The Working Group for Electronic Data Interchange is a network of healthcare-related people who have formed to design policies for information management. A system must be created to use a special code rather than a name and social security number to label patients so personal information is not attached to their medical records.

The actual implementation and definition of the requirements set forth by the Health Insurance Portability and Accountability Act (HIPAA) have been areas of great diversity and confusion. The Administrative Branch of the federal government is supposed to oversee HIPAA and the result has been a changing definition of HIPAA processes. The healthcare industry has attempted to remain knowledgeable about the changes to keep in line with HIPAA by forming groups of people who are designated to keep up with the ever-changing HIPAA regulations. Oftentimes, healthcare organizations use outside companies to create their computer systems and must rely on the company to protect information by HIPAA standards. The communication that occurs between the healthcare organization and any outside agency accessing the information must also be protected by HIPAA standards. Every person within the healthcare organization and those people otherwise associated with the organization must be trained and knowledgeable about HIPAA standards to ensure they are following the standards in every aspect of their job.

## Information security threats

Natural disasters can occur at any moment and preparation for potential issues that could cause the loss of protected information within a healthcare organization must be a part of a healthcare company's plan. Information that is entered into the computer should be copied and kept away from the place of input so if a disaster occurs, the information can be retrieved. The frequency that the information will be copied should be predetermined and scheduled. The education of management and personnel within an organization is critical. Everyone should be walked through exactly how they should react in case something unexpected should occur. A plan should be developed for who is responsible for retrieving the copied information and how it will be input back into the system once the system is fixed. A computer virus, or bug sent through a computer system which is meant to destroy the system, must be prepared for. Many companies offer programs to detect and stop viruses from harming the system. Time and money should be spent in the careful selection of the very important virus protection programs.

Ensuring specific information is guarded against security risks is important. The computers must be protected from people who are unauthorized to access the information on the computers, which is covered by physical security. An unauthorized person may attempt to steal a hard drive or computer terminal, so these items should be safeguarded. Information contained within the computer should be protected from unauthorized users through the use of technical safeguards. A unique set of characters created by the system's users should be required for entrance into the computer system. If input information is especially private, data encryption or changing the input information into code only understood by internally designated personnel, may be necessary. The healthcare organization should keep a file of when and by whom system information is accessed or modified. Education of all employees regarding security expectations is essential so everyone knows what they are supposed to do and the consequences for noncompliance.

## Evolvement

Medical care has become more efficient and successful over time. People within the field have developed new treatments for disease and new ways to prevent disease. As a result, technology has been created to assist in medical care and has evolved with medicine. Older demographics, or the fact that people live longer as a result of better medical care has led to advancements and greater use of medical care. The increased cost of healthcare has resulted in the need for government intervention. When people cannot afford coverage, they look for government assistance. The government could not afford to pay for the gaps in coverage and political dissatisfaction was the result. The solution has been to create set rates on medical procedures so medical providers cannot overcharge consumers and consumers can in turn take financial responsibility for their healthcare coverage--a system known as managed care. The goal has been to achieve the best medical service with the least amount of money being wasted.

**Hospitals**

The role of hospitals has evolved over time. They were first meant to provide medical services to groups of people in a central location. As technology has improved to meet the demands of medical practices, hospitals are needed to house technology so procedures can be performed that require longer term care than a physician's office can provide. Hospitals can be owned by the government, businesses that are paying for the hospital without making money, and companies that are paying for the hospital to make money. Government hospitals are research based and partner with schools or are designed to meet some need within the general public. Government hospitals cannot be tied to a church. Some businesses buy hospitals, called not-for-profit hospitals, which are meant to help a community but are not meant to earn the owners money. Some groups of people or businesses purchase a hospital to make money and they are called for-profit hospitals. Big hospitals located in big cities are the most commonly used hospitals. The effectiveness of the people overseeing a hospital's operation is the greatest indication of the success of the hospital.

The people or companies who own hospitals have frequently decided to merge their hospitals together. When 2 or more organizations decide to bring their hospitals together but remain as separate owners, the arrangement is called an alliance. All owners have to agree on major decisions and getting agreement can be an insurmountable task. When 2 or more organizations come together to create a new and separate hospital, a health system is created. A health system has one decision maker who is responsible for the needs of the organization as a whole, rather than the separate parts that created it. Most hospitals are health systems. Health systems often come together to provide service to the most amount of people over the largest distance possible. The result is that one organization profits from an entire area or many areas. For example, a major city like Houston, Texas requires many different hospitals. Memorial Hermann owns many hospitals in different parts of the city, thus providing services for most people living in and around Houston.

## Primary care and specialist physicians

As the medical field developed and more treatments for specific areas of the body were created, physicians, called specialists, were needed who could be experts in different aspects of the healthcare field. Some doctors know a little bit about all areas of the medical field and are called primary care physicians. If the primary care physician cannot effectively treat a patient, they send them to an expert in the specific problem called referral specialists. Specialists earn more than primary care physicians and the majority of specialists have a specialized certification in their field of work. Most doctors have their own facilities where they administer services. Some merge together to form practices with many doctors, typically because they are all part of an insurance company's HMO list of doctors. Some doctors and hospitals work with insurance companies and are paid a set rate for each treatment and at the same time work with managed care payment. They are referred to as physician-hospital organizations.

## Health insurance

The 3 main sources of medical coverage are employer-sponsored health insurance for working adults and their families, Medicare for the elderly who qualify and Medicaid for the less fortunate of society. Without the use of one of those sources a person can buy coverage from an insurance company privately or can go without coverage. Some companies and Medicare pay for medical coverage for their employees and those covered by their plan respectively. Insurance companies, like Blue Cross and Blue Shield can be used to represent the business or Medicare to make sure doctors are paid correctly. The insurance company is thus a middleman, or intermediary, between the company and physicians. The insurance company also serves as a representative of the large company to ensure the company is paying the best price for medical services, which is detailed in the Medicare Act Preamble. The use of insurance organizations as a middleman between medical providers, the people they service, and the company who pays for the medical care leads to greater expenses for all involved. A doctor may be prone to adding in unnecessary charges or procedures to get more money for his or her services. The patient will not be as quick to question the procedures because he or she is only paying predetermined co-pays. The price of insurance however increases over time. Strategies have been created by businesses to overcome these problems. One strategy is to require the people working for them to pay for part of their insurance coverage. Co-payments and deductibles have been set up to increase the amount a patient must pay towards his or her medical services. Doctors have been limited as to how much they can charge for a procedure. Insurance companies have created lists of doctors for users of the insurance to choose from called HMOs and PPOs. Some insurance companies pay a predetermined amount based on what is determined to be wrong with the patient, called provider risk sharing. To help with medical progression and to ensure excellent care is being provided, pay for performance (P4P) plans are used.

**Clinical systems, microsystems and patients**

Clinical systems oversee the groups of people formed to work together on a particular case or patient. People needing medical care often have problems that require seeing a variety of physicians and offices to care for their ailment; clinical systems help all people involved function together in the best possible way. These alliances of physicians and caregivers are known as microsystems and must rely on help and oversight from the leaders and other departments within their organization. Microsystems need communication support and help to determine the best ways to make a positive medical experience for both the people needing medical service and their loved ones. Because the same patient may see several different doctors each with their own diagnoses and treatment options, some level of communication must be maintained in order for the patient to receive the best possible care. People involved in the microsystems should monitor this communication and make necessary alterations.

**Healthcare organizations**

Because government regulations reduced the amount of money medical providers could charge for services, coupled with the fact that the government could not afford to pay for people without insurance, medical providers have had to respond by creating strategies to make money. Medical providers do this by creating criterion to evaluate their services against goals called benchmarks and by weighing themselves against others providing similar services. Many banded together in a central location with other providers offering different medical services to create healthcare organizations (HCOs). Centrally locating physician's means they can share expenses and work together to create cost-saving strategies. HCOs are convenient to patients, acting as a one-stop shop for medical services. Some diversity exists in the success of HCOs because their success largely depends on variables such as the type of customers within the population they service and the HCO's location.

All people will need to visit a healthcare organization (HCO) at some point in their lives. Some are financially capable of paying for the medical care while others are not. The population and government must share in the cost of providing medical services to all people in need. It is important that healthcare organizations exist to reduce the spread of diseases. Easy access to medical facilities is a reason for people to locate in an area and jobs are available at an HCO. HCOs strive to provide the best and most affordable medical services. Benjamin Franklin articulated these reasons for needing hospitals in a population in 1760. These are the same reasons HCOs have formed and are successful in today's society.

Healthcare organizations (HCOs) have to listen to the needs and wants of their customers. Consumers want good care at a reasonable price. They want their physicians to be knowledgeable in their service and fair in their pricing. Consumers want every area of their healthcare needs to be covered by insurance and their physicians. A HCO that is well-managed will listen to the needs of their consumers and make the necessary modifications to meet the patient's demands. The care provided will not only include what is necessary while a patient is at the doctor's office, but also include the needs of the patients in the aftermath of their recovery. A well-managed HCO will make an effort to help patients maintain wellness and avoid illnesses. The departments within a well-managed HCO will communicate and work together effectively for the good of the patients. The HCO will combine what is known to work well within the healthcare industry while creating new strategies for the success of the medical providers and the patients.

Healthcare organizations (HCOs) are open systems which can be defined as a group of people who are affected by and communicate with those people whom they represent. An HCO uses their assets both concrete and abstract to care for a group of people. Every part of the system must work together for an HCO to be successful; in turn, the HCO can only be as successful as its weakest component. In order for the HCO to function, products--both human and nonhuman--and money must change hands, which are interactions known as an exchange. Some groups of people are required by contract to interact with a company and they are called exchange partners. People who own stock or have a financial tie to an organization are a group of exchange partners known as influential. They can give or withhold resources in order to accomplish a personal goal. An HCO represents the medical providers and the people needing service and must balance the needs and wants of both groups.

**Customer exchange partners**

A healthcare organization (HCO) provides service to people needing medical care and the HCO must be responsive to the needs of this group of exchange partners. People who are ill or need medical care want excellent care in an adequate setting and want their medical providers to listen to their concerns and the concerns of any loved ones who are present. HCOS must be able to act as representatives for the people who need medical care, protecting their interests and acting on their behalf. The groups, including insurance companies, Medicare and Medicaid who pay the HCOs are exchange partners with the HCO. HCOs must consider the groups' needs and represent the groups and themselves in a mutually beneficial way. HCOs should understand that those paying for medical services want to do so by paying the least amount necessary for quality care. Companies who pay for health insurance for their employees often use an intermediary or buyer to shop different insurance companies for the best rates and service. The buyers are another group of exchange partners.

The Joint Commission on Accreditation of Healthcare Organizations (JCAHO) and the America Osteopathic Association are 2 agencies that ensure hospitals are following required guidelines. Their oversight is required by insurance companies and other people who financially fulfill patient's obligations. The government has similar agencies that ensure that financial transactions are completed within set guidelines. In order to make alterations or create a new hospital, the hospital must frequently obtain a certificate of need from the state government. Companies who pay medical benefits on behalf of those in need use quality improvement organizations (QIOs) to ensure that the financial transactions are completed fairly for both the insured and the company paying for benefits. Because anyone in need of medical services can access a hospital, child protective services and other agencies acting on behalf of populations of people in need have interactions with healthcare organizations. Although most HCOs do not pay community taxes, they are responsible to the community's expectations and must communicate with and comply with community standards.

A healthcare organization (HCO) has many people who work together to bring the organization success. The happiness of the people contributing to the organization is important for an HCO to consider. Some people are paid to work for the HCO, while others work for free; both groups must be respected so they will work at their optimum ability. When several people come together for a common purpose an associate organization is developed. Internal organizations will communicate the needs of the group with the HCO. The medical technology and materials needed by an HCO come from outside vendors. The HCO needs money to get the merchandise and often makes deals (called strategic partnerships) with outside companies that are mutually beneficial to the HCO and outside company. Because the type of care varies from patient to patient, a physician may need to refer the patient to another physician or care facility. Sometimes an HCO will make deals that benefit both the HCO and the source of their referral. Government oversight of HCOs requires HCOs to give certain private information to the government when requested.

**Stakeholder contributions**

The groups or organizations financing an HCO, or stakeholders, must be satisfied because they are responsible for the growth or failure of an HCO. If physicians choose not to be a part of an HCO, the HCO has lost revenue and cannot grow. If people using an HCO's services are dissatisfied and discontinue use, revenue is lost. The more people involved in the HCO the better its success. If there is discourse between stakeholders, the HCO must remain neutral, listen to both sides and come up with the best possible solution that will appease all involved in the problem. The HCO relies on word of mouth of people they service to spread amongst the places and institutions they frequent. The fewer friendships or networks the HCO forms in the local population, the less influence the HCO will have and fewer customers will use their services.

**Measuring success**

A valiant effort has been made to oversee if HCOs are achieving excellence while servicing patients. The Joint Commission on Accreditation of Healthcare Organization and the quality improvement organization were both formed for this purpose but neither has produced long-term positive results. Lawsuits have become a common way for people to seek monetary compensation for poor care. Unfortunately, there are many frivolous lawsuits that have impacted the desire for physicians to take risks that may be beneficial to patients. The National Quality Forum (NQF) has been a more successful tool in the oversight of HCOs. The group evaluates the HCO based on a detached perspective focusing on what the physician is actually doing and comparing that to the end result. Those getting better results are scored higher and subjectivity is removed from the equation. The Agency for

Healthcare Research and Quality can be contacted to see how different HCOs are doing, thus allowing people choosing an HCO to see the results.

**Financial transactions**

Financial support is needed for a healthcare agency to be successful. Debate has existed over who should provide the financial support and how much financial support is necessary. The following questions apply to the debate. Do physicians make enough or too much money? Should patients have to pay more for medical services? Do insurance companies profit too much from premiums? Appeasing all involved in the financial needs of the HCO is difficult because layoffs or degradation in quality may occur. The prospective payment system (PPS) was designed to determine a fee that would be paid per sickness, referred to as a diagnosis-related group (DRG) by Medicare for patients entering the hospital. Doctor's fees were determined by the relative value scale. Insurance companies followed suit and set limits on their payments. Because the various groups adopted the same strategy, HCOs had to accept the terms to remain competitive.

**Moral standards**

There are many people who work in a healthcare organization (HCO) in many roles, such as those that service patients and those who serve administrative roles. An HCO's success depends upon the morality of the people involved in the organization. Employees must value people and want to serve every individual regardless of the patient's appearance or belief systems. Every person should be shown the same level of esteem and dignity. The people working within an HCO must strive to provide the best care possible. After an illness is cured, the person relieved still wants some level of service from the HCO and this fact must be considered for an HCO to be successful. The fact that the healthcare industry is constantly changing and new and better techniques can be applied to meet the demands of change, should be known by those working for an HCO. A successful HCO will communicate its desires and expectations to potential employees and hire people based upon their agreement with the HCO's standards. Positive rather than negative reinforcements should be used to gain compliance from employees regarding the set standards.

## Future goals

The Institute of Medicine's Committee on Quality Healthcare in America looked at the current state of the healthcare industry and developed guidelines of expected behavior for the future. The protection of patient's health at a more efficient rate is an expectation. Use of the appropriate type of medical care the first time a patient visits a medical provider is another goal. This calls for less subjectivity in patient care from physicians and an increased use of evidence-based medicine. Giving the patient all options available for the treatment of his or her medical condition and allowing them to make an informed decision without pressure from a physician is another goal for future HCOs. HCOs should be available for patients at their hour of need. Education of patients on preventable illnesses should be part of an HCO's planning and budget. HCOs should begin considering that both poor and rich people need care and should be able to provide affordable plans so all can access and use their facilities.

In order for the future of healthcare to run more smoothly, effort must be made on the part of healthcare organizations to develop strategies that will avoid the need for complex and expensive medical procedures. As people live longer, they will need medical care at a greater rate and for a longer period of time. Effort must be made to educate people and encourage people so that they will make better choices when it comes to health. Cigarette use and other harmful activity must be discouraged and those who are already addicted should be helped in quitting. Maintaining a healthy weight should be emphasized. It is much more cost effective for a healthcare organization and the population to avoid medical procedures if possible and maintain healthy lives instead. Both curing diseases as well as developing strategies to help people avoid getting diseases is the goal of an integrated health system (IHS).

## Mission statement

A healthcare organization (HCO) is constantly changing its strategies so it can function at its optimum capability, which is known as a continuous improvement strategy. A mission statement outlines the fundamental goals of the HCO and declares how it will uniquely strive for excellence within the industry. After reading the mission statement, the reader should understand why the HCO formed. The virtues of the HCO should be detailed in the mission statement. The mission statement should be visible and known by employees within the organization and accessible to those people visiting the HCO. The mission statement should become the standard for the HCO and all changes and modifications to the HCO should be weighed against the mission statement. Employees and anyone else doing business with, or representing the HCO in any way, should be in compliance with the mission statement.

In order for a mission statement to be fulfilled within an HCO, a strategic system must be followed. A strategic system requires the HCO to respond to the changing climate of the healthcare setting. The people within the organization, those receiving medical service from the organization, and businesses which interact with the organization, will react to changes; the HCO must measure the changes against the mission and make adjustments as necessary. Plans need to be developed to make sure the HCO is in touch with the spoken and unspoken concerns of the people responsible for its financial success. Once the mission is established, plans of action must be defined in a business plan. The business plan should define objectives that can be measured and monitored for success. When and who will be tasked with completion of the items within the business plan should be described. Many HCOs are forming alliances within groups of providers who perform tasks related to a common disease, or service lines, as part of their business plan. The doctors cannot perform medical procedures without available facilities, the facilities are maintained by people providing clinical support services, and the interaction should be addressed in the business plan.

Every successful organization will put its overall goals and broad ethical standards into a mission statement. In a healthcare organization (HCO), the governing board creates the mission and all modifications to the HCO are measured against the mission to ensure compliance. When considering modifications, the board first takes a look at a big picture of the healthcare field to find areas that need improvement. Based on the information gathered, the board can consider new strategies that help their HCO become more competitive while remaining in line with the mission statement. The board then considers cost, in terms of both human and non-human capital to complete the strategy--which is referred to as resource allocation decision making. There are immediate costs and costs that will continue for however long the project takes to complete. If all of the information gathered favors a project, the HCO will proceed.

**Continuous quality improvement (CQI)**

Because the healthcare organization (HCO) is dynamic, customer service must constantly be monitored and made better, which is a theory known as continuous quality improvement (CQI), created by W. Edwards Deming. How well the HCO is functioning and CQI must be analyzed by quantitative analysis and comparison to set standards or benchmarks. A HCO cannot be successful financially or in any other way without bringing in people to use its services. Developing strategies to maintain the people already using the medical provider and developing strategies to bring more people into the practice is another aspect of CQI. It is important that those who work within the organization feel they are valued and know that their voice is heard. Employees need to know that their opinions can lead to new processes, which is a concept known as empowerment. Open communication between business leaders and employees is fundamental in employees feeling empowered in the workplace.

## Shewhart cycle

As various aspects of business are analyzed, solutions need to be created to make the healthcare organization run better. Performance improvement teams (PITs) are formed to create new and better business tactics. "Plan Do Check Act" (PDCA) or the Shewhart cycle is a system that helps PITs form new ideas and carry them out. The Plan step involves the investigation of current work process to find any areas of inadequacy and the determination of reasons for the inadequacies. The Do step requires the PIT to brainstorm on better ways of completing the task that will overcome the inadequacies ultimately choosing a best practice. The Check step requires the PIT to set in action its new plan and determine if it actually works in a real setting rather than just in theory. The Act step requires the PIT to bring the new idea to actualization and move on to a new process improvement.

## Technical and logistic support

Clinical systems need technical and logistic support from the HCO to function properly. This support includes detailed and up-to-date information on the people needing medical services. The physicians providing patient care need to be informed on best practices or protocols that have been accepted within the industry. The patient's billing and payment status is important to know. Another area of support needed by a clinical system from an HCO involves the personnel involved in the system. The best workers are desired and the system relies on the HCO to find and keep quality employees happy. State of the art technology is used by the best clinical teams which are supplied by the HCO. People who must visit the healthcare organization should have easy access to the building and should be provided with a comfortable atmosphere both of which are provided by the HCO. HCOs use people who form responsibility centers to determine when there is a need for improvement and to discover and implement process improvements.

**HCO management**

Leaders are needed to oversee an HCO in many ways. It is up to management to find areas that are in need of improvement within their healthcare organization. Top managers need to know how their HCO is impacting the population where it is located and should spark communication with community leaders to determine the impact. On a smaller scale, department managers can determine how their HCO is doing by asking questions of employees and customers. Because the details of patient's records are so important, leaders within an HCO should consistently review how information is input and make sure employees are knowledgeable in the process and its importance. Senior management should be involved in creating education plans for their department managers to implement and department managers should use the plans to educate new employees or existing employees about new developments. Both senior management and department management should be involved in developing strategies to make the HCO better. Both levels of management should be involved in making sure the people within their organization are working together in a positive way and should be involved in overcoming conflicts when they arise.

The people who work as managers within a healthcare organization (HCO) must be educated in the industry as well as with the specific department he or she is overseeing. The owners count on their managers to identify problem areas and be intelligent enough to fix the problems. The education level of management is typically a master's degree or doctorate. Supervisors are accountable for their department's performance and many HCOs use a multi-rater review to grade the supervisors every year. The manager of the supervisor who is being evaluated, other supervisors at the same level and people who work for the supervisor all have input. The National Center for Healthcare Leadership creates standards for good managers and the performance of healthcare supervisors can be weighed against these standards. After reviewing the results of the supervisor's review, the HCO will design a personalized development plan, which is a plan of action to improve the supervisor in areas of need. Because there is turnover in management of an HCO, some supervisors are chosen by the HCO to fill upcoming positions in a succession plan.

Effective managers are vital to a healthcare organization's (HCO's) success. Education on how to be an effective manager is necessary for a manager to be successful. Managers need to be taught how to listen to their employees as well as their supervisors and implement new ideas, rather than just providing a sounding board for problems. When a new procedure or practice is passed down from the board for implementation, the manager must be taught how to effectively transition his or her staff to accepting the new organizational path. Management capabilities can be taught and a successful HCO will spend money and time training their managers. Effective managers will make sure that evaluations are completed on employees and on the organization fairly and without bias so the HCO can be improved. The manager should protect the integrity of the evaluation system for the HCO while removing any personal feelings from the process.

Many situations will arise where a healthcare manager will have to implement a new strategy that may be unpopular with the staff. For example, the governing board may decide that the HCO needs to save money by limiting the amount of overtime available for nurses. The nurses may deem this as unfair. It is up to the manager to hear both sides and make both sides as happy as possible. One way for a manager to encourage a positive conclusion is to treat every person involved with the same respect regardless of his or her position. Management should also make decisions based on facts rather than emotions. If necessary, the manager must fire the employee to resolve the conflict. Managers should have the ability to act as a mediator in disputes and look for areas that need to be communicated more clearly. Sometime managers may need to approach a situation by explaining to their employees that the board has come to a conclusion and nothing will change the decision, so acceptance is the only strategy.

## Governing board

A group of people oversee the entire HCO and are called a governing board. Governing boards are necessary in making sure everyone contributing to the HCO is working together effectively so goals created by the board for the HCO are achieved. The governing board acts as a liaison between the HCO and everyone contributing to the HCO. Without customers, or stakeholders an HCO cannot function and it is up to the board to make sure both groups of people are happy. The overall purpose of board members is to make the most money possible for the owners of the HCO and they are measured by how much money they can make for the organization. If an HCO is designed not to profit, the board members, called trustees, are responsible for ensuring the HCO is financially successful enough to continue to operate. Board members are responsible for oversight and support of the HCO. They make

decisions on which departments and who should receive financial support. Some would argue that board members should provide financial support to the HCO so they have a personal stake in the success of the organization.
The board must consistently check to ensure the HCO is functioning properly and well. One way the board checks quality is by watching how well each department does with its goals set forth when the HCO's financial plan or budget was created. If a major area of concern arises, the board will alert the department head to develop a strategy to fix the problem. The board is not meant to fix it themselves, but rather ensure that it is addressed. To make sure that the information received by the governing board is true, audits are conducted within the HCO and the board ensures the audits are completed to their satisfaction. At times, audits are requested from companies not related to the HCO especially in areas of monetary oversight. The goal of using external auditors is to make sure the HCO is covered legally from discrepancies and to make sure auditors within the HCO are being honest and doing their jobs correctly. All major business opportunities conducted between the HCO and outside companies are overseen by the board.

Beyond its administrative and budgeting duties, an HCO must also oversee and maintain the quality of the medical services provided for by their organization. This is an important duty, because failure to provide quality care can result in legal action. Quality is monitored by outside agencies like the Joint Commission on Accreditation of Healthcare Organization (JCAHO) and government agencies. The board allocates monetary resources to quality care, creates regulations for its employees called medical staff bylaws and is involved in ensuring quality leadership is hired within their organization. The oversight of hiring medical staff by the board and holding applicants to strict standards provides the HCO with quality employees. The board members are supposed to be neutral and should hire based on merit rather than personality or other political factors. If a problem arises with the medical services provided to a patient, the case is investigated by fellow medical providers through a process of peer review. The board hears the results of the peer review and ultimately decides if culpability applies.

**Board members**

A potential board member should be able to weigh information carefully and without bias and form decisions based on logic rather than emotion. Board members should be able to maintain the best interests of the HCO and its owners at all times. They must be motivated by doing a good job rather than how their position can further their personal lives. The board members must know the people their HCO will provide service to, including their needs and wants from the HCO. Not only do the board members need to know the medical profession, but they must also be skilled in business and negotiation. Board members must be available to serve when needed. The board members should have prior positive experience and be well thought of by people who have worked with the members in the past. A variety of types of people--including those with a variety of skills and those with different backgrounds--should be on the board. Different genders, races and ages should be considered based on merit.

When a spot is open or becoming open in a governing board, many boards have the power to pick a replacement and these boards are referred to as self-perpetuating boards. Sometimes the people who own the HCO or work within the HCO can select board members. The leaders within the board are nominated and accepted by the board members. Most boards have a group of people who seek members to work on and lead committees and seek people to be on the boards. The committees are called nominating committees and they pick candidates for board approval based on the number of board members needed. There is a designated time frame board members can serve on a board, 3 or 4 years being the standard. Some boards require their members to invest monetarily into the HCO. Most board members are not paid for their service, but serve for the experience and dignity the position holds.

Chief executive officers (CEOs) communicate frequently with and advise board members although they are not typically members of the board. The CEO of an HCO is chosen by the board, so the CEO and the board have a close relationship. The CEO is the board's eyes and ears within the organization and the board relies on the CEO for accurate and essential information. Problems can arise if a CEO in any way tries to advance his or her own agenda rather than protecting the HCO as a whole. For example, a CEO may advise the board that a certain department needs funding for a project. If the board gives the money and the project fails, a CEO may try and hide the failure to protect his or her personal interests. Choosing a trustworthy and honest CEO becomes vitally important to an HCO. Doctors hold seats on most boards within HCOs. They know best what is going on in the healthcare field because they work in it every day. The doctors on the board must be careful to represent all doctors as a whole rather than address problems or make improvements that will help the doctor serving on the board personally.

The limited number of physicians on the governing board must represent the needs and important issues of the staff as a whole. The HCO's goals and overall evaluation of the way the HCO is functioning is looked at every year to determine areas for potential improvement. The physicians on the board and other physicians who are held in high esteem have input in the board's meetings. All fields of medicine are represented in a hospital and each specialty has different needs. It is important that all fields are represented in developing the strategic plan for the HCO. Some specialties need more money to buy up-to-date equipment that is necessary for quality care. The physicians therefore need input in the budgetary process of the HCO. If an HCO is contemplating providing a new clinical service for patients, the physicians can provide input into how the implementation will affect the HCO both financially and otherwise. Because a physician can make payment arrangements with a patient that includes personal rather than insurance payment, an agreement must be made between the HCO and physician about possible nonpayment that will affect the HCO. Physicians should have input into the types of payment arrangements they want to accept.

Board members are not full-time employees of the healthcare organization (HCO). Many have separate careers from their duties on the board. Leaders within the HCO are tasked with helping the board be successful. One way in which department leaders can help the board is by providing the board with data that relates to their department. The board needs the HCO's leaders to be their eyes and ears within the organization. The communication between the supervisors and the board should be in writing and should provide all essential information that a board needs to make informed decisions. The data provided should be free of bias and should be fact based. Because a board member does not necessarily work within the healthcare organization it governs, supervisors are responsible for the instruction of board members on relevant material. The supervisors within an HCO become the face of the board. They must represent the overall goals and ideals of the board to the customers and employees they come in contact with.

**Legal issues**

A board can be sued by outside parties. The board as a whole is typically the target and the board has lawyers to represent them in case of a lawsuit. Because most board members are part of the medical community they have significant ties to the healthcare industry. For example, a person may serve on the board for an HCO while working full-time as a CEO of a medical supply company. Legal issues can arise over conflicts of interest. If the hospital was looking to switch medical supply firms, the board member should not use his influence over the board to make sure his company is chosen. Personal investment and work information should be stated by each board member to avoid potential problems. In HCOs which work for the needs of the community rather than to make money, legal issues can arise around how they spread their wealth amongst the community they serve. This should be a non-biased process and is governed by inurement rules. When two separate businesses become one--called consolidation--or when an organization working for the community, becomes one that makes money from the community (called conversion), legal issues may also arise.

**Chief executive officer (CEO)**

The people who are on the board of an HCO are typically temporary and the board job is not their primary source of employment. The board makes determinations together but their plans must be set into action by one person. A chief executive officer (CEO) is chosen by the board and the individual chosen is the main representative of the board. He or she leads the employees within the organization and is the contact point for those people interacting with the HCO outside of the organization. The CEO must be knowledgeable in every aspect of the HCO because he or she is the communication source between the board and the remainder of the HCO. A person who fulfills all of the requirements is hard to find and the board must choose carefully. The board should compile a list of traits they desire from a new CEO including specific qualities, education and experience.

When a CEO is chosen, the board should clearly explain its expectations in an employment contract. The contract should not only detail the board's needs but should also explain how the board will evaluate the CEO and how the CEO will be paid for his or her services. If for any reason the relationship fails, the contract should explain how it can be voided. Legal problems may arise so this part of the contract should be clear and understood by both the board and the CEO. The board and CEO should work together to determine areas of improvement for the HCO that will occur within the next calendar year. The contract should clearly discuss how the CEO will be rewarded for working for the HCO. The salary and other compensation should be competitive so a good CEO will remain within the organization. Bonuses for meeting and exceeding benchmarks may be part of the CEO's contract.

**Balanced scorecard**

Each year the board of a healthcare organization will meet and determine goals for major areas affecting the overall success of the organization. The board details each area in a balanced scorecard so they can visually track the HCO's success throughout the year. Each area on the scorecard is rated for success and the end result is a clear representation of each quarter's successes and failures. The amount of money an HCO is making is a standard area that is tracked by boards. When the board allocates the budget, it does so on the basis of the different categories on the scorecard. When setting the goals on the scorecard, the board reflects on the HCO's past performance, other HCOs' performance, market performance and areas that are of priority to the HCO; how the money will be allocated, or the budget is created, and the board makes modifications and eventually agrees upon the HCO's budget. Each department is given an operating budget allocating how its resources will be used.

Departments within a healthcare organization (HCO) have goals they must meet and their performance is tracked in an operation balanced scorecard. One area on the scorecard reflects how much the HCO is being visited--known as demand for service. The number of clients an HCO is seeing and how that number has increased or decreased is a measurable area on the scorecard. Another area in the scorecard measures how many of all the people in the surrounding community of an HCO are using the particular HCO being measured. The HCO may look like they have seen a good number of patients for a year, but if their competition has seen twice as many, a problem is identified. Another area on the scorecard measures if the proper treatment is being administered regardless of the patient's request. The ability for an HCO to respond to needs of patients is another measurable area.

Resources are a measurable area on the operation balanced scorecard. One part of the area of resources is known as physical units. Management must project how many employees are needed at a given time, at what times equipment can be used, and how much inventory is on hand. All of the areas are tracked in physical units. The price of physical units is determined by a standard industry amount placed on what is used by the healthcare organization, which produces costs--another part of resources on the balanced scorecard. The number of resources and how well they are being used is part of the resource condition measures portion on the scorecard. Another area on the operational scorecard involves employees and is called associate resources. The specific qualities each employee possesses that will benefit the organization are tracked in an area known as supply measures. How well the qualities are being matched to the organization's needs is measured. Another measurable area under associate resources is called development measures and involves assessing employee's skills to make sure they match with the needs of the organization and the search for educational opportunities when they apply. Satisfaction measures are used to determine how happy the employees are with the healthcare organization they are working for. How happy an employee is, is directly tied to how long they will work for a company and their attendance and their happiness is analyzed through loyalty measures.

The operation balanced scorecard has an area called "outputs" which is designed to evaluate the production of a healthcare organization (HCO). An important area to consider is how well the organization is supplying service to patients requesting care. The measurement is based on the result rather than the number of requests. How well requests for service are met with actual service provided is measured and the result is known as productivity. Clinical support services are part of every procedure and each is an expense for the provider. Activity-based costing is the term used to describe the analyses of the expenses. Hospital space and certain equipment can generally be quantified in a set number, meaning they are fixed resources. When a fixed resource is not used, it is not making money for the HCO. The amount of time any/all resources are not being used is measured.

The operation balanced scorecard has an area called "quality of care" which is meant to evaluate the level of care the healthcare organization (HCO) is providing. When a person enters an HCO, they do so with a problem that needs diagnosis and treatment. The clinical outcomes portion of the scorecard tracks a person's end result or outcome of receiving care. Clinical outcomes can be tracked by recording when treatment goes wrong. For example, if a 50-year-old patient goes in for a routine heart procedure, has complications and dies, the result would be tracked. The hospital can track all heart procedures or death rates in patients over 50 or any combination of areas that can be measured to reduce mistakes. Another way to track clinical outcomes is by asking the person who received medical care if they feel it worked. Tracking the patient's success from a fact-based evaluation of results, typically through the use of a paper called an SF 36, is another way to measure clinical outcomes. Lastly, the HCO can track where a patient resides after they are cared for thus evaluating the patient's level of independence.

**Hiring staff**

A group of people called a planning staff determines how many physicians for each department in a healthcare organization (HCO) will be required and drafts its findings in a medical staff recruitment plan. The board must agree with the plan for it to take effect. The board considers how many patients will be requiring the services so the doctors can work at their craft, if there is sufficient monetary resources to pay the physicians and if it is worth it to the HCO to spend the money. The board investigates doctors on their staff to make sure they are providing excellent medical care and the board ultimately appoints physicians based on their credentials for a set period of time. The board maintains oversight of any outside agreements made between the HCO and groups outside of the organization. The board and the HCO lawyers review written agreements and decide whether or not the HCO will enter the agreement.

### Subsidiary boards

A healthcare organization (HCO) often has many different healthcare centers under its umbrella. Each center can have a separate governing board, called a subsidiary board, that communicates with and report to each other and to the main HCO board. Subsidiary boards are important because they are located within the community they serve and therefore know their patients and their marketplace best. It would be difficult for a governing board located in one city or state to make effective decisions for a healthcare location in another city or state. Because the healthcare centers under an HCO's umbrella can differ in services they provide, subsidiary boards ensure that people who are familiar with the specific types of services being offered are represented on the board. Having boards for separate organizations makes it easier if the separate healthcare organizations decide to become one in a joint venture because each HCO involved has a board representing its unique interests. The various boards allow for certain tax benefits because the organizations are functioning separately.

In order for subsidiary boards to function properly, they must have the freedom to make decisions and oversee their healthcare organization separately from the main board of the HCO. The main governing board of the HCO must have oversight of each of the subsidiaries and their oversight is detailed in their reserved powers. Reserved powers are powers that the main board maintains to control its subsidiaries. The overall goals of the HCO are important to everyone affiliated with the HCO and the governing board of the HCO makes sure the subsidiaries are in line with the goals. If one subsidiary has a dispute with another subsidiary, the board decides how the issue will be overcome. The governing board of the HCO is in charge of the purchase or release of assets, how money will be dispersed among the organization and managing the subsidiaries.

### Successful boards

A governing board that is full of ideas and process improvements, but never makes the next step in implementing their ideas, is as ineffective as a governing board that never has a new idea. When strategies are created, the governing board must determine when the strategies will be implemented and follow the timeline as much as possible. If issues arise, the timeline should be adjusted, but movement forward towards completion must be the overall goal. Strategies cannot be implemented without the appropriate knowledge to do so. The board is involved in improvements they initiate, but are also responsible for government-regulated activity. In order to complete a task correctly, research must be completed before the project even begins. Board members and their employees handle the task of gathering appropriate information. Because there are multiple areas that must be considered with great detail by the board, the board needs to take time on each important issue. If their careful investigation is not required, the board can approve these items in a consent agenda.

**Standing and ad hoc committees**

A governing board does not always have the time available to carefully research and consider every issue that comes before them. They must assign some of their responsibilities to other people or groups of people who can make the appropriate effort--which is a system called delegation. Standing committees, such as an executive committee, are often given responsibilities from the board. The standing committees should be given detailed tasks to complete and timelines for completion to ensure they are in fact performing the function they are assigned. If a standing committee is not specialized in a certain area that must be addressed, the board can form an ad hoc committee for a designated timeframe. The ad hoc committee is tasked with investigating a problem and finding solutions for the governing board. The opinions of ad hoc committees are almost always implemented by the board, because the committee is created for a particular function by the board.

**Evaluating a governing board**

Some of the actions of a healthcare organization are governed by law and a good board will be knowledgeable about the law and make sure their organization is participating in authorized activity at all times. A successful governing board will provide continuing governance education (CGE), which means they will make sure the people working within their HCO know the most up-to-date and most highly recommended medical practices and procedures. The governing board should promote participation from all members when the board comes together because each person on the board is valuable and should be heard. If individuals on the board are involved in any private activity that could conflict with the best interest of the board, the individual should be required to disclose the information. A separate group of people disassociated with the board should be formed to maintain oversight of the board and resolve any conflicts that arise within the board. The board as a whole manages the chief executive officer and this duty will not be overlooked by a successful board.

### Service excellence

Employees who feel respected and are treated well work harder for their employer. Managers within a successful healthcare organization (HCO) recognize and foster good relationships with the employees they manage--a theory known as service excellence. Making an employee happy within an HCO and creating an organizational culture means providing them with the materials and education required to do their jobs correctly. All people within an HCO and customers of the HCO must be treated fairly and equally by management. Employees should feel secure in bringing up concerns so management can evaluate issues and take action when necessary. Healthcare management should never lie to employees or ignore inquiries made by employees. Management should refrain from making subjective decisions when possible and instead rely on scientifically proven facts. The leaders of an HCO should act like they want their employees to act. If they are upholding positive standards, most employees will follow the management's lead.

### Evidence-based continuous improvement culture

A healthcare organization (HCO) can never remain stagnant. The healthcare field changes and the atmosphere created by management within an organization must reflect their acknowledgement of change, which creates an evidence-based continuous improvement culture. Management should create objectives, use financial resources to obtain the objectives, let their team know how close they are to achieving an objective, and recognize the employees' roles in achievement of an objective. Employees should feel confident that if they are working hard towards a task, management will do everything possible in overcoming problems that may arise. The team must feel like management cares about their project as much as, if not more that the team itself. When process improvement teams (PITs) are created to resolve a problem, they are led by performance improvement councils (PICs). The PIC should manage the progress of the PIT and should aid the PIT whenever necessary.

## Accountability

There are many departments within a healthcare organization. Management of the people working in each department is essential and a supervisor is assigned to each group to oversee activity, making it a cybernetic system. A cybernetic system is one that is overseen by either a human or non-human to ensure it is functioning correctly. The supervisor of a healthcare organization (HCO) cybernetic system must detect areas that are not in compliance with expected results and make necessary changes to regain compliance. If the supervisor in charge of a workgroup is not meeting the HCO's goals, action will be taken to get the supervisor in compliance so the supervisor is accountable to the corporation as a whole. Each level of people within an HCO is accountable to somebody, all the way up to the owners who are accountable to themselves. A supervisor of the information technology department should not be accountable to a supervisor of a surgery center. The 2 departments are unrelated and the supervisors are the same level of management. Different areas in the HCO will have an accountability center that knows their processes and can manage the group successfully.

## Communication needs

Part of a successful healthcare organization's (HCO's) plans should include strategies to make communication successful. Data and other information are continuously exchanged within departments and many times the information needs to be transmitted to others, both inside the organization and outside of the organization. Each level of the accountability hierarchy has a designated role in the communication process. Most communication that affects the HCO as a whole is conducted through the computer. The Internet is used to communicate with external customers while the company's Intranet is used to communicate within the organization. A patient's personal information is typically input into the computer creating a patient record. The patient's payment status is tracked on an accounting ledger. The information is sensitive and must be protected whether it is kept in a computer system or in paper files.

## Epidemiologic planning model

The governing board must assess the need for growth of their healthcare organization (HCO). In order to determine how many people within the population surrounding an HCO will need to use its facilities for inpatient or outpatient care, an epidemiologic planning model is used. The model is used to determine what types of doctors will be needed based on past use. The model divides the actual usage of a hospital for either a particular procedure or number of customers in the previous year by the total number of the particular procedure or number of healthcare customers of the industry as a whole within a designated community for the previous year. If an HCO cannot compile the data itself, it can buy the information from an outside vendor. An HCO can look at the results of past models to see if they were indeed accurate. This can help the HCO decide if a change has occurred in the marketplace and to identify specific types of people who need healthcare services.

**Strategic partnerships**

The medical field is complex and there are many areas of specialties. Not only do the many different types of patients need to be served by people familiar with how to care for each unique issue, but lab tests are required and the office must operate clerically. There are few HCOs that can provide every service requested to the extent that will meet or exceed the patient's needs. The leaders within the HCO must oversee the organization and find areas where cooperation with doctors or other external offices is necessary. Doctors who are knowledgeable in a variety of areas of medicine, known as primary care providers (PCPs) sometimes partner with HCOs to either work for the HCO or work with the HCO. If an HCO does not provide a specific service, it may partner with specific providers who specialize in the area of need.

Most HCOs do not have an environment conducive to extended care, so they may work with long-term care providers. Because the people in the community that the HCO serves are important contributors to the HCO, the HCO forms partnerships with local groups that provide community service. An HCO must be kept clean and the equipment must remain in good condition, so many will hire outside companies to perform the task. Materials are needed for an HCO to provide medical care and an HCO will often enter into extended agreements with vendors that include discounts on bulk orders and better supplies. The need for educated people to work in the healthcare industry is always high and many HCOs will give money to local educational institutions for students in the healthcare field. Most HCOs are paid through the use of insurance, so they will partner with certain plans for the mutual benefit of both the insurance company and the HCO.

**New patients**

In order for a healthcare organization (HCO) to maintain success, it needs patients. Patients want to know that the healthcare organization they choose will provide a safe and pleasant environment. Many insurance companies offer their customers choices of healthcare organizations, creating a competitive atmosphere. The competitive environment means that leaders of an HCO must communicate to the population that surrounds the HCO the reason they should choose their organization over another similar organization. Accidents and lawsuits will occur surrounding an HCO, so the leaders must find a way to maintain confidence with their organization. The media is a communication avenue where leaders can reach a great number of people with a positive message. Speaking and partnering with groups that serve the community is another way to strengthen an image. Making patients happy so they tell others of their positive experience is the most powerful way to bring in customers.

## Mesh model

Main leaders in healthcare organizations maintain oversight and communication with multiple departments and large numbers of people. There is a chain of communication that leads to the governing board in an accountability hierarchy, but many healthcare organizations are under a mesh system. This means that one person, who is the supervisor, has communication over many different channels, and the various departments have unique organizational goals that may be different from the main organization's goals. The mesh system leads to the creation of groups within the organization called service lines. Service lines reflect the needs of their specific patients rather than a generic goal. Objective measurements are used to evaluate service lines and if a service line is not functioning properly, it can be replaced. Service lines understand how easy they can be replaced and in return, function better to avoid it.

## Clinical outcome measurement problems

Because patient's information is now frequently kept within a computer system, the information can be manipulated and tracked easily. The reports that can be generated provide management the opportunity to measure almost anything they can imagine. The problem with having a wide variety of reports available is that the healthcare organization (HCO) can draw incorrect conclusions from the results. For example, the HCO may be measuring how well a new type of pacemaker works for heart patients. The results may show that 75% of the people who got the pacemaker had further heart problems and may decide the pacemaker is ineffective. The problem could be that half of the patients receiving pacemakers were also smokers, which really caused the further complications. When creating areas of measurement, all factors should be accounted for, including a patient's medical history, and considered before drawing a conclusion.

**Measuring quality of care**

Quality of care can also be tracked by how well the organization is in compliance with accepted standards by the healthcare industry as a whole, through the use of process quality measures. Some programs like Medicare fine HCOs for noncompliance with industry standards of care. Best practices can be applied to any area where the HCO is failing. A step-by-step instruction of treatment has been created by CMS, which is defined by the patient's diagnosis or symptoms. The National Quality Forum has created a more general approach, which is based on best practices for the industry as a whole rather than based on a specific medical problem. They list 30 procedures that should be followed to ensure the patient is well cared for in a secure environment. Another agency, the Malcolm Baldridge National Quality Program, has established a list of areas where the provider's competence can be tracked to determine the level of care being provided. Working equipment and qualified staff are needed to provide quality care to patients and their availability is tracked on the operational balanced scorecard under the heading of structural quality measures.

**Surveys**

The operational balanced scorecard tracks how happy the person receiving treatment is with the care they received. The happiness of the people visiting a healthcare organization (HCO) can be determined by questioning the people upon departure or upon completion of care. The HCO can create their own surveys or external companies can be used. The benefit of using an outside company is that they have standard questions that are used industry wide and thus management of one HCO can compare its results to another HCO's performance. Generic measurements of satisfaction can be also be used that apply to any organization, not just healthcare. SERVQUAL has created this type of measurement system that asks questions regarding broad areas like reliability and empathy. Ultimately, the HCO needs to discover if the patient would revisit the HCO and if they would recommend the HCO to others. Many times a patient is required by insurance to get a referral from his or her doctor; or they just value the opinion of a doctor they know regarding another physician. How happy the doctor is with the service provided by the referred doctor is tracked through the use of questionnaires. Any other person who has received service from an HCO is frequently surveyed for their happiness with the HCO.

**Clinical performance**

Clinical performance is a term used to describe how well a healthcare organization (HCO) is caring for patients, while taking into consideration the level of resources the HCO has at its disposal. A community hospital may not have as many resources available as a private hospital, but clinical performance is based on the performance of each in providing medical services using what they have available. In order for clinical performance to be considered good, the healthcare organization must follow the needs of the population it services, thus allowing the people served to establish the level of economy. Good clinical performance requires the HCO to listen and follow the recommendations of the physicians providing the medical services. All departments within an HCO are interrelated and must work together for good clinical performance. If there is a weak link among the departments, the clinical performance will suffer.
Part of clinical performance includes developing strategies to help people avoid getting sick and developing strategies that encourage good health. Most healthcare organizations (HCOs) exist to help the people they service, so prevention of disease and the healthy lifestyles of people they serve are fundamentally important to the HCO's cause. People see healthcare providers when they need care and will listen to the healthcare provider. Even though preventing disease will stop the people from needing future healthcare services, HCOs continue to make prevention a priority. There are 3 types of prevention of illnesses: primary, secondary and tertiary. When a shot is given to stop a person from getting sick or any action is taken to avoid an illness, primary prevention is applied. Once an illness has already been established in a patient, secondary prevention is used to lower the negative effects caused by the disease. In order to stop a sickness from happening again or to avoid unnecessary side effects of the disease, tertiary prevention techniques are followed. When establishing protocols, the HCO should make sure that prevention and healthier behavior is part of the long-term plans.

Clinical performance has to be monitored for efficiency and possible improvements. The Leapfrog Group, National Quality Forum, Institute for Healthcare Improvement (IHI) and the JCAHO all recommend quality healthcare practices that will help improve clinical performance. The JCAHO created National Safety Patient Goals. The Goals listed include the following: ensuring that people receiving medical care are properly identified so mistakes in care can be avoided, ensuring that medicines that could have potentially harmful side effects are administered correctly, avoiding medical mistakes, and ensuring that healthcare providers are discussing patient problems openly and frequently. Pay for performance (P4P), or paying healthcare providers based on positive results stemming from their patients care, has been used by many health insurance companies to help facilitate good clinical performance. If physicians are paid to provide better care, the patients will benefit from the P4P programs. The insurance companies are hoping that P4P payments will encourage a reduction in costs associated with incorrect care.

**Decision model**

A clinical quality improvement program involves creating best practices for healthcare. The theory is that money will be wasted on experimenting with different treatment programs, so best practices should be used the first time. In order to achieve clinical quality each patient's symptoms must be considered and the most efficient treatments must be determined. For example, if a patient comes in with chest pain, the doctor must decide the cause of the problem. The physician can do this based on symptoms or order an x-ray. An x-ray is an expense and the price of the x-ray must be weighed against the positive result of having it. If an x-ray is ordered when it is not necessary, good clinical performance is not achieved. The more complex the procedure is which a physician is considering, the more time the physician should take to weigh the price of the service against the benefit. Mathematical probability equations can be applied to determine the benefit of a complex procedure.

By applying a decision model in the process of determining the best medical course of treatment, the patient can feel secure that whatever treatment is used will be beneficial and necessary. The patient can also feel secure that the doctor has not just based his or her treatment on a test, but rather has applied logic and weighed options before deciding the best course of action. Applying a decision model ensures that the physical and monetary price of a medical procedure is completely necessary for proper treatment. If the best treatment is done the first time, the patient will have an easier time during the procedure and in recovery and will typically not have to repeat or try a different procedure. Many times there is more than one way to treat an illness, but applying the decision model assures that the best treatment is chosen. If a patient has a medical problem, quick treatment is often necessary and important. Applying a decision model in the beginning will avoid unnecessary time being wasted on incorrect treatments.

## Healthcare providers and continuous improvement

Because all medical care is completed by people, the people administering care are a major factor in the process of providing quality care. Healthcare provider's development is part of the continuous improvement process. Healthcare providers should be encouraged to take a proactive role in determining new and fresh ways of maintaining good clinical performance. The medical providers should be involved in brainstorming sessions to determine better methods of performance, what schooling they need to stay abreast of changes in the medical field, and rewards for acceptance of any changes that are made. The result of the process will be a new and better path for clinical activity. Healthcare providers should approach continuous quality care with the mindset that process can always be made better and each area of the process should be investigated to decide if a better way can be applied. The person's need, who is receiving the medical treatment, is most important and the good of the whole HCO should be valued.

## Clinical expectations

Clinical expectations are standards for what resources, both human and non-human, will be required in completion of a medical procedure or patient care. These standards are set and accepted by the medical profession as a whole so patients, insurance providers, and physicians all know in advance what they will need to complete a patient's treatment. Clinical expectations are part of the following 3 groups: functional protocols, patient care plans, and patient management protocols. Standard practices followed by healthcare providers in the completion of routine medical care are grouped under functional protocols. Functional protocols are used frequently and are typically memorized by providers. A functional protocol is a step-by-step process by which a treatment is carried out. If a part of the protocol is not followed, the results can be detrimental to the patient. By following a functional protocol exactly, the steps can be traced in case a problem arises. The healthcare organization should clearly define situations where a specific protocol should be applied and when it should not be. The protocols should be monitored occasionally for possible improvement.

Patient care plans are one group of clinical expectations. A unique patient care plan should be created for every individual who visits a healthcare provider. Once a physician listens to a patient's symptoms, he or she should begin a plan of action based on applying known medical treatments, or management protocols, to the patient care plan. The plan should clearly state the desired outcome of a treatment plan. What exactly the physician plans to do to treat the patient, or component activities, should be detailed in the patient care plan. There should be a place where details of care can be written down in order to communicate with other potential medical providers. The patient care plan should have a timeline with expected dates of treatment. There should also be a place in the plan where evaluation of the plan for effectiveness can occur and redesign can be possible.

**Patient management protocols**

Protocols that are established by profession and accepted by a healthcare organization (HCO) as a whole are called patient management protocols. Clinical practice guidelines are established by medical experts and the HCO can choose what guidelines they feel are best suited for their organization. The National Guidance Clearinghouse (NGC) compiled many of the various clinical practice guidelines that can be weighed for selection by an HCO. Guidelines listed on NGC provide details on symptoms and what steps a medical provider should follow when certain symptoms are discovered. Where the information came from is also listed within the NGC. Management must respond to the demands the guidelines require. The goal of using patient management protocols is successful treatment which is measurable, based on the results of using the guidelines. If the guidelines chosen by the HCO do not give the expected results, the HCO may choose another guideline to follow.

Applying developed protocols to patient care in the healthcare industry is standard and management and healthcare workers find following established standards acceptable in providing quality care. The employees are trained based on protocols and they therefore follow the established guidelines. If a healthcare provider lacks experience in a certain area but needs to care for a patient, he or she can use protocols to provide care. A healthcare provider can deviate from part of the protocol if that will better suit a patient's needs, but he or she should document the deviation. If a deviation is proven to be more effective than the guideline itself, the protocol can be reviewed and adapted. Functional processes are made better by the use of protocols because there only needs to be one right way of providing standard medical care and, once established, everyone can follow the same procedure and everyone will require the same training and equipment.

Accepting a protocol as the standard for a healthcare organization (HCO) requires careful consideration of all potential protocols available. An HCO cannot rush to pick a guideline, but should meet as a group and determine what will happen once a protocol is accepted. Different opinions from experts who will use an established guideline should be heard and considered. A new protocol will have to be prepared for and the new guidelines taught to the medical staff, both of which should be considered by management before accepting a new protocol. Because people have unique medical problems, protocols cannot be rigid or unchanging. Management should monitor the effectiveness of protocols and change them when better guidelines are established or new medical technology is developed. If a medical expert decides that a specific patient needs different care than the protocol defines, he or she should have the ability to use his or her judgment to determine the best course of action.

**Preventive healthcare strategies**

Strategies must be established for a healthcare organization (HCO) to reach the population they service when it comes to leading healthier lifestyles to avoid sicknesses. The goal of the HCO is not to see people in the community for preventable illnesses and because of this the HCO must somehow communicate the message outside of the walls of the organization. By using a decision theory model, the HCO weighs the price of care for an illness against the expenses used to help the person avoid the illness. The HCO looks for ways to provide the community with services to prevent illnesses that make the most financial sense to the organization and that can affect the largest number of people--a process known as optimization of preventive activity. The HCO reduces its expenses by finding and using tests that generate high accuracy, because if a preventive test is wrong, the HCO wasted money.

Because there are so many preventative healthcare strategies available, the healthcare organization (HCO) should establish a plan for which strategies they will adopt and will be most effective for their organization. The HCO must consider the people the strategies they enact will affect and determine which will be most effective and important to that group of people. This opinion of the people the primary and secondary prevention strategies will affect should be weighed against the costs to the HCO. If a plan can be easily implemented, affect a large group of people, and the cost of implementation is low, the plan should be ranked as first on the list for implementation. The HCO should look for groups within the population they service that will help spread the prevention plan to as many people as possible, thus reducing the cost of communication for the HCO. There are many community groups with similar agendas to the HCO, including helping the general public and the HCO and these community groups can work together to better the community as a whole.

## Problem areas

The role of a healthcare organization (HCO) is to ensure that patients are treated based on evidence, that people seeking healthcare are satisfied and happy with their experience, and that physicians enjoy doing their job personally and professionally. Managing the numerous physicians and other healthcare providers employed by an HCO is difficult because there are so many people in several different locations. The fact that many doctors are experts in a specific area rather than general practitioners compounds the problem, because each physician has a special way of providing care based on their expertise. The way physicians earn their income adds a problem area for the HCO. If a physician refers a patient, the referring doctor sometimes gets paid for the referral. If paid for each treatment provided, many physicians will provide more care than necessary to make more money. If limited by an insurance company, the physician will make less money. The conflicts in how physicians are paid results in physicians putting less effort into helping patients avoid getting sick, because they get paid more when they provide healthcare services rather than preventing them.

## Arranging the personnel

One model that has been used to arrange the medical staff within a healthcare organization (HCO) occurs when the HCO maintains a medical staff. The medical staff works under structures provided by the HCO but are not paid by the HCO and still work individually for themselves. The HCO can monitor the physician's results, allow the physicians to make recommendations for the HCO and provide training to those on the staff. The problems with the system arose because primary care physicians began to maintain private facilities and no longer needed the hospital to provide care for patients. Patients who needed more complex care were referred to experts in their condition who could use the HCO on a case-by-case basis. The medical staff was not required to pay the hospital to use the facility and could not under law discuss payments. Another model occurs when the HCO actually hires and pays a medical staff. A drawback is that the HCO is responsible for the salary of the physician as well as providing equipment and facilities so the physician can do his or her job effectively. Because the physician knows he or she is earning a salary regardless of how many patients he or she sees, members of the medical staff are not as customer oriented as private practice physicians.

Medical staff is arranged based on common goals, but the arrangement of the staff varies by healthcare organization (HCO). The staff is arranged to provide excellent service in the most cost beneficial way. This includes ensuring that patients are treated well while resources are not wasted. Allowing people to make payments that they can afford will help an HCO be able to service a large number of people who may not have paid anything for healthcare services. The education and experience of doctors hired by the HCO is very important in providing excellent care. The HCO should arrange staff so that it can ensure the doctors are happy in their work. Salary and other financial incentives must be comparable to other organizations. Promotion and education opportunities should be provided for the doctors. The HCO must be effectively sustained economically and socially.

**Privileging**

Doctors are evaluated based on a system called privileging. The goal of privileging and credentialing is to ensure physicians are qualified to provide medical care. Once qualified, the physician can make medical decisions and provide service to patients. The NCQA, JCAHO and legal cases have determined what is required of doctors to become privileged. The bylaws of the privileging agreement were set forth by doctors who agreed upon guidelines that all doctors must follow. The physician organization through the bylaws determines standards for care, salary, and other requirements that can be legally upheld if a source of conflict arises. Once a doctor decides to become a part of a physician organization, they are rewarded with privileges as detailed in the privileging agreement. These privileges include the physician becoming part of the organization sometimes referred to as attending physicians. Physicians within the organization are part of a review process by which their medical colleagues evaluate their fellow physicians in cases where patient care is questioned.

The privileging agreement details the relationship between the physician and patient. The independent physician-patient relationship portion of the agreement is meant to define the primary relationship between the medical provider and the person he or she is providing treatment to, understanding the relationship takes priority over the relationship between the medical provider and healthcare organization (HCO), a methodology known as agency. The doctor is expected to provide the same level of service whether being paid by the patient or the HCO. A major goal of any HCO is to monitor its performance and make modifications that will better the organization and doctors working for the organization are held to the same standards. This is detailed in the continuous quality improvement and peer review section of the privileging agreement. The peer review portion describes how medical colleagues will evaluate each other.

A group of people, called a committee, who can evaluate physicians fairly and without bias is formed to review who will receive privileging credentials. Privileging is an important responsibility and the most trusted physicians should be part of the committee. The bylaws set forth should be followed in picking who will be credentialed. Following bylaws ensures there is no special treatment afforded to any physician up for review. An executive is in charge of overseeing the meeting and ensuring rules are followed. The doctor being evaluated has input into the process. He or she can view the same information the committee views and make written statements about the information. If there is a dispute between the committee and physician, attorneys for both sides should be present. To ensure that all people in the medical community can be made aware of someone who has his or her credentials removed, the Health Care Quality Improvement Act created in 1986 requires the removal to be reported to the federal government.

The privileging committee bases their review on 4 set standards. The doctor must have up-to-date training, proper certification, and ongoing experience in his or her field. The doctor must demonstrate that he or she is doing his or her job correctly and according to set protocols established for his or her area of expertise. The physician must have the general public's interest in mind and serve the people seeking medical attention as effectively as possible. The doctor must not do harm to or abuse other physicians or the people he or she serves. If the doctor meets all of the requirements he or she will be privileged. If the doctor is not effectively treating patients, his or her credentialing can be taken away by the healthcare organization (HCO).

Certification, or the path to receiving certification, is a general requirement to become a privileged member of a healthcare organization (HCO). Some HCOs require doctors who work in a specific area of the healthcare industry to have a certification unique to their field of work. If the HCO cannot provide the necessary support of a specialized physician's work, they may not privilege the doctor. The HCO may require the doctors to service a set amount of patients so their abilities remain well honed. If a doctor wishes to become privileged in another area of practice, he or she must prove that he or she has received the training necessary to perform the extended function. Because privileging can be general or specific, there is some debate as to how much it is necessary to have experts work on cases. Doctors in general practice feel they can treat most patients where specialists feel they are necessary to providing the best care. Another area of concern is that if a specialist is the only person privileged to perform care to a specific patient group, he or she will be the only person who can profit from caring for the patients, which excludes general practitioners or other specialists.

**Conceptual planning model**

Healthcare organizations (HCOs) must balance the number of doctors they have working within their facility against the number of total physicians needed by the community. If there are too many doctors, some will go out of business because there are not enough patients to service. If there are too few doctors, the patients will not get quality care. HCOs use a conceptual planning model to determine the number of physicians required. The model multiplies the number of people in the community who will potentially have a medical problem by the number of illnesses or treatments and divides that number by number of treatments completed in the previous year. To determine how many potential doctors need to be hired, a model is used that takes the previous problem's solution or the number of doctors required and subtracts how many doctors are already working for, and will continue to work for the HCO.

**Physician supply plan**

A well-managed healthcare organization (HCO) will evaluate how many doctors are needed to successfully service a population of people and create a physician supply plan. This plan also makes sure that there are not too many doctors servicing the same customers, which can cause them to make less money. Specific areas of the healthcare field that see many patients in a given year should be analyzed annually to determine how many doctors are needed and those who see few patients should be analyzed to determine the necessity of keeping the areas of specialty. Because healthcare is dynamic and constantly changing, the HCO has to consider what circumstances may affect future demand. The governing board has the ultimate say on how many doctors will remain on staff and how many will be brought on staff. The HCO should also decide how many patients will be referred rather than serviced by the HCO and how these referrals will impact their overall income.

**Physician recruitment plan**

The physician recruitment plan requires careful consideration by the healthcare organization (HCO) because the HCO will have to pay any physicians that it recruits.

If the estimations of physicians needed are incorrect, the HCO loses money. The HCO has to estimate how many people will need specific types of care, how many and how much care their current physicians will provide, and what specialty physicians will be needed to provide patient care. Groups of doctors meet, debate, and come to agreement on how many and what specialties of physicians to recruit. Once determined, money is spent by the HCO to find good doctors and provide incentives that will make the doctors want to choose their particular HCO. A recruitment group decides on the qualifications required of the person they are seeking, how much they will be paid, where they will find potential recruits, and ultimately who they will choose.

## Education

A healthcare organization (HCO) that employs a staff is responsible for ensuring they are receiving up-to-date training and education. Each HCO follows unique protocols that are constantly updated and part of the education process requires teaching the staff how to follow set protocols. Training about business-related functions is important for an HCO to provide to its physicians. Putting a physician through training requires paying for the training and paying for the time the doctor must spend away from treating patients, known as opportunity cost. The JCAHO has stated that HCOs should provide their doctors with monthly training to ensure they are performing at an expected level. Not only doctors, but other healthcare staff should be continuously trained. Postgraduate education is often paid for by an HCO for new doctors called residents and fellows, who are trying to become specialized in a specific area of medicine. The Accreditation Council for Graduate Medical Education (ACGME) evaluates and accredits postgraduate schools.

## Physician-hospital organization

Physician-hospital organizations (PHOs) were created as a partnership between physicians and hospitals and, in order to get physicians to participate, healthcare organizations provide monetary and other benefits that entice doctors to join. Because many insurance companies are now charging a fee per service rendered, called capitation, the practice has required the healthcare organization to come up with new integrated healthcare models that will earn money for the organization and physician while maintaining quality care. One strategy is to help patients control their illnesses so they do not end up hospitalized for long periods of time. Another strategy is to have a patient's care, both initial and ongoing, in one healthcare facility. HCOs have spent money developing computer systems so hospitals and doctors can communicate and share data effectively. Another model encourages patients to be involved in the direction of their healthcare.

**Communication between physicians and the HCO**

Doctors often have different viewpoints and agendas that are specific to their area of expertise. The bylaws should set forth how to handle disputes, including the creation of committees to make general decisions for the healthcare organization (HCO). If physicians do not feel like they are being heard, they may leave the HCO; so communication is very important. It will not benefit the HCO to ignore the needs of doctors; but a strategy that includes going to the physicians and asking what concerns they have, is a better, more proactive approach. It is less necessary to form committees, create plans, and document activity if an atmosphere of trust between physicians and the management of the HCO is formed. An HCO can create this relationship by taking the time to talk to the doctors within their organization and respond to their needs whenever possible. Some doctors within the HCO are on the governing board and they provide the closest link between healthcare management and the actual issues that practicing doctors face.

**Physician payment**

Insurance companies have set payment schedules that they follow for patient care. These are negotiated either with individual doctors or in the case of a patient-hospital organization, a large group of doctors. The insurance company and physicians are limited in how much they can charge in hopes of making more money by the Office of the Inspector General of the U.S. Departments of Health and Human Services. The Current Procedure Terminology (CPT) is a system where physicians who are not under a specified medical plan enter the medical procedures they perform to determine an acceptable price. If there is a service not in the CPT, a doctor can keep the extra money. A withhold contract exists when an HCO keeps part of the fees earned by a doctor and only releases the portion of fees if the doctor meets quality goals. Another way physicians get paid is through the use of capitation, where they are paid based on a set number of patients they provide medical care for. Sometimes a plan will not cover a procedure or type of care and physicians can be paid separately for the care.

Doctors get paid from a variety of sources and in a variety of ways. If a physician organization hopes to keep quality doctors on staff, they must develop strategies that help physicians get paid as mush as possible. Contracts regarding a physician's income are diverse. One contract deals specifically with how much the HCO will pay the physician to be on staff. Another contract an HCO can negotiate is with insurance companies. The more insurance companies that approve their members to use a facility, the more the HCO and physicians will get paid because their will be a higher volume of patients. An HCO will provide many administrative functions for the physicians so the physician saves in the cost of maintaining records. Physician organizations can negotiate the sale of an individual doctor's office so the physician can begin working for the physician's organization. A physician's organization can enter into a contract with the physician to invest with the organization so both can profit.

**Home care and family training**

The health of the population as a whole is a top priority for healthcare organizations (HCOs). This means providing services for people who are not sick in order to maintain their health. Providing long-term and full-time healthcare is expensive and many people simply cannot afford it. One strategy an HCO employs to prevent a person from having to live in a full-time care facility is training people who are relatives or non-professionals on how to care for a person with an illness or disability. They can be taught how to help a patient get better if possible. If a person can be cared for away from a medical facility, the cost is much cheaper. Home care is thus another way an HCO can provide service to a patient.

**Resolving conflict**

Physicians who are part of a physician's organization often face conflict with the organization. Conflicts arise around the fact that doctors have to follow certain rules set forth by the physician organization but may feel that another way is better. The doctor may want to work beyond the organization's guidelines if they feel their patient will benefit. Many physician organizations encourage compliance by streamlining conflict resolution. If the doctors understand that whenever conflict arises the organization will react in the same manner, they can more easily accept the resolution. The physician can remain confident in the fact that protocols are developed with the patient's interest in mind and that as long as the HCO is following protocols, quality patient care is being delivered apart from any agenda the physician's organization may have. The physicians can rely on standard ethics committees to ensure that the organization is overseeing compliance. The physician organization attempts to come to resolutions that are equitable to everyone whenever possible so no one doctor is treated better or differently than another. If a physician still disagrees with a resolution, he or she can enter into an appeals process to fight the decision.

**Community healthcare needs**

Most healthcare organizations (HCOs) have the resources and thus the responsibility to oversee the population it services, to discover areas where more healthcare services are needed, to ensure people are happy with services received, to ensure excellent care is provided and to correct any areas that are lacking in excellence. This ensures that the HCO is meeting the needs of the population it serves and can make alterations to the services it provides to meet the needs of the community. The HCO has to gather a great deal of information to get accurate and complete data so that it can determine how comprehensive its services are compared to services in other comparable market areas. The Behavioral Risk Factor Surveillance Survey can be accessed to find out state-wide healthcare information which the HCO can use to compare itself against. The goal is not so one HCO can compete against another. The goal of the information is to make all HCOs better for the community. Some HCOs will partner in data collection or use a community agency like United Way to gather the information.

One healthcare organization (HCO) cannot provide for all of the medical needs of a community. Even if the HCO employs every type of specialist available, they will not be able to employ enough people to meet the entire demand of the community. The HCO should meet with other service providers and make sure all community needs are met. The role of an HCO in meeting with different types of medical service providers and agencies is difficult because there are many agendas represented. Not all want to talk to an HCO and some even feel that the HCO has the same types of customers and therefore could be taking customers away if the agency decides to work with the HCO. These issues cannot deter the HCO from its goal to make sure the community needs are provided for, but the HCO must realize potential problem areas and have a response when the issues arise. The HCO can use money to accomplish its goals by either partnering with an agency to provide a needed service or by giving money to an agency for the same purpose.

**Case management**

People who have disabilities but can still manage to live away from long-term healthcare facilities and people who have other problems that require long-term care need help in finding resources and healthcare. Healthcare organizations (HCOs) should provide the resources. Many patients cannot afford to pay the huge medical bills that result from the need to see a physician or specialist on a regular basis. The people still need medical care and it is up to HCOs to make healthcare possible through the use of case management tools. The HCO can oversee a patient's care and find cost effective ways for the patient to find healthcare. Most patients with ongoing problems need to see a variety of types of doctors and HCOs can use their relationships with agencies to provide for each person's unique needs.

**Community support for preventable diseases**

Healthcare organizations (HCOs) have the resources and responsibility to create community programs that will lead to the avoidance of primary preventable diseases. If there is a shot that can help a child or adult avoid getting sick, an HCO should provide the shot, or immunization to people within the population it services. Any concern that affects the community and can be prevented by an HCO educating people to get out of or avoid a potentially dangerous situation should be acted upon. The people with the greatest financial need in the community are often the most difficult to reach, but require prevention services the most. The HCO should use its alliances formed within the community to reach as many people as possible because they all have the same goal, which is to help people in need. If these people are not reached with preventative healthcare, many will not be able to afford necessary medical treatments once they acquire a preventable disease.

**Secondary prevention of diseases**

Once a person acquires a disease, they need medical treatment and the sooner treatment is given, the more effective it is. Community support from healthcare organizations (HCOs) is needed to find these people and help them avoid spreading the disease. The HCO must figure out ways of locating these people, which is part of providing secondary prevention. An HCO can find people by providing free testing to the population it services because once they are found, the HCO can help provide needed healthcare. Many people exposed to a potentially deadly disease need to be sought out by an HCO because they do not willingly seek medical treatment. The HCO must create strategies to find people who are at high risk for disease and get them into a facility to be tested. The HCO should help preventative programs like Narcotics Anonymous (NA) in any way it can as a responsibility to the community.

## Ambulatory agencies and housing issues

The healthcare organization should provide ambulatory agencies with any help possible, because they are servicing the population the HCO also services. As part of its community-assistance strategy, the HCO should help programs that bring healthcare to patients, especially when the patients cannot afford to or otherwise do not have the means to visit a healthcare facility. Although HCOs are not directly involved in ensuring patients have a place to live, if the facilities are inadequate or patients become homeless, the HCO industry will clearly be affected. The HCO should communicate and help agencies that provide support for people with housing problems to come up with ways to fix problems that result from the inability of a patient to find a place to live.

## Long-term healthcare availability

Healthcare organizations (HCOs) do not have the space or financial capability to keep people in their hospitals for long periods of time. There still remains a need for these types of living arrangements and HCOs should help patients find either care that can be delivered to their place of residence or a nursing home. The best way for an HCO to help the population it services is to find the best quality and least expensive long-term care. If the HCO finds a long-term healthcare provider that is needed by the community but is not providing good care, it must react. The HCO can open a business that provides better services, can tell patients to use only the providers that provide excellent service, thus removing business from poor ones, or can offer financial or other support where a need prevails. The HCO will be spread into different areas providing different types of care for a variety of people and it can sometimes become difficult to manage each of the healthcare facilities.

## Accounting

The financial management portion of a healthcare organization (HCO) is responsible for locating and tracking any financial dealing that has bearing upon the HCO--which is called transaction accounting. There are many transactions that affect an HCO financially, including employees, furniture for a waiting room, and technology. Every item has a cost and transaction accounting keeps track of every item and cost. Most paper money is collected by an HCO when employees are providing medical assistance, or service to patients and their loved ones. The people working for the HCO and the equipment bought that cannot be sold, but is necessary to the HCO, make up resource transactions--which are also tracked in transaction accounting.

The information is input and displayed in cost ledgers. If the transaction occurs within the HCO, it is referred to as a general ledger transaction. The cost associated with each type of transaction can be determined either by a concrete method or an educated guess based on previous experience.

A healthcare organization must show how it is spending the money of its owners, people it owes money to, and anyone else who has interest in the financial dealings of the HCO. Financial accounting is the process by which the information is provided in terms that the interested parties will understand. The compiled information is presented in a balance sheet, or report showing the overall financial situation of an HCO. How much money has been made by the HCO or any money losses are also presented in a report. Where money has been allocated is another report provided to interested parties. The last report shows how much money is left in different areas of the HCO. The governing board must frequently review these reports because they are responsible for the financial oversight of the HCO. The HCO is responsible to the population to give accurate information and will allow their reports to be audited by an outside source to ensure accuracy. Revenue accounting is based on how much money the HCO collects for its services--rather than how much is charged--providing net revenue. Money the HCO earns from sources other than the people it cares for, called non-operating revenue, is also tracked.

Some healthcare organization's (HCOs) expenses do not change and are known as fixed. Some expenses depend on circumstances, like the number of patients being serviced, and are known as variable. Some fall somewhere between the two and are known as semi variable. Managerial accounting evaluates expenses for their category or type and compares them against different forms of pricing. Managerial accounting determines how much money is needed to accomplish accounting goals. Another role of managerial accounting is to determine if it would be cheaper for the HCO to create supplies in house rather than going to a vendor for purchase. Part of managerial accounting includes evaluating the functions of the HCO to see if there are areas for improvement which could save the HCO money. Information must be gathered for analysis which is specific to the pricing and financial information of the HCO.

**Cost control guidelines**

Managers must have the ability to analyze financial data in order to create strategies for making the financial portion of the healthcare organization (HCO) more successful. Managerial accounting is the process by which financial information is gathered in a way that managers can perform their oversight. Managerial accounting involves looking at a price paid for every item and examining to see if the price paid follows certain guidelines. One guideline involves determining if money output is within the budget--which is a process known as control. Another guideline, comparability, requires the determination of whether or not the price paid is competitive and within the standards of the HCO. The last guideline, or profitability, is meant to determine if the price paid is low enough to leave the HCO with some money, or profit, so that it can meet future objectives.

**HCO budgeting**

A budget is an estimate of how much money will be spent for the budget period--usually created annually in a healthcare organization (HCO). Short- and long-term goals cannot be achieved without necessary funding and budgeting allows the HCO to determine areas of need. One area of the budget is called the operating budget. The operating budget determines expenses for the various departments within the HCO and usually includes only expenses in the direct control of each department. Another part of the operating budget is called aggregate costs or those expenses not specific to a department, but that are relevant to the HCO. Another part of the budget includes money that each department is expected to receive called revenue budgets. Financial budgets project how much money the HCO will make and cash budgets track how much money comes in and goes out of the HCO in a period of time. The part of the overall budget that tracks how much money the HCO will spend is called the new programs capital budget.

Healthcare organizations (HCOs) have clinical departments that attempt to provide excellent service while working within a budget. To do this, a new clinic's management must first look at the employees who must be available for the clinic to provide service to its patients. The salaries paid to employees are required and therefore are fixed and are direct, because the employees work specifically for the clinic. The second cost area is associated with the medical supplies needed for a clinic to operate. These expenditures must be tracked and must meet the patient demand. Management must avoid unnecessary waste or surplus, which is dependent on the amount of people using the clinic. Another way to keep the cost down is to find vendors who charge the least amount while maintaining quality. Another area of cost concern is that associated with sending out for tests or other clinical support services. Management must weigh and determine in what situations it is best to outsource clinical support services.

Once cost data has been compiled, it is presented by the controller to the healthcare organization's (HCOs) management. The reports should take into account the budget and report for the same period and timeframe as the budget. The information should be up-to-date. They should provide the number of and cost of everything included in the reports. The reports should only include relevant information so it can be easily understood. The reports should be analyzed to show areas where benchmarks are clearly not being met. The reports should be presented and accessible to all people in the organization to whom they are relevant. The information should be presented consistently to all members of the HCO. Activity-based costing (ABC) is designed to price activities as they are being completed so that a more accurate number is achieved.

Management attempts to determine what areas of the healthcare organization will need money when creating a budget. There is a give and take between departments' wants and needs. Management must determine how many customers will request service, how many customers each department is actually servicing and how much everything costs. The areas of the HCO that receive the most business are analyzed to determine how many patients will be seen in the future. This is based on previous experience and management's analysis of market trends. Once the number is calculated, the HCO assumes that all of the customers coming in to the HCO will be provided with medical service, so management can use the same number of patients being seen as the number of patients receiving service. The cost of resources is determined by how much was paid in the past and applying normal increases based on the market. The cost of production, including employees and facilities, is also estimated. Some budgets can be changed based on circumstances that cannot be concretely defined ahead of time and are called flexible budgets.

### Financial planning

Part of financial planning for a healthcare organization (HCO) includes the creation of a long-range financial plan (LRFP). The strategic plan is analyzed to determine how much money will be brought into the HCO and how much money will be output, which is detailed in the LRFP. Large loans are typically 30 years long and must be factored into financial planning. Ratio analysis is used to compare how much money or capital is leaving the HCO versus how much is coming into the HCO. Ratio analysis is used to determine if the interest paid and other fees related to borrowing from an outside source is worth it, areas where savings can be found and made, how much actual money is needed to pay off people who the HCO owes money to, and to determine if the consequences of any decisions dealing with money are worth the potential consequences.

Because financial planning requires estimating and analyzing information many years in advance, changes will occur and part of financial planning is anticipating changes. All companies go through normal highs and lows and money loses purchasing power year after year which must be accounted for in a financial plan. People move in and out of the market, other healthcare organizations (HCOs) take customers, and medical equipment gets better—all of which affect how many customers an HCO has. Government regulations and insurance changes will also affect financial estimates. To make a long-range financial plan (LRFP) complete, all of the situations should be considered. Without all of the information, it is impossible to count on the results of the financial plan. The governing board counts on financial managers to provide them with complete and accurate information so they can make an informed decision.

A main goal of a strategic plan and financial planning is to make the healthcare organization (HCO) money, and a plan must be created to determine where to allocate the money that is being made. Some of the money made must be put back into the HCO to keep it functioning well and keep equipment and technology competitive. The HCO attempts to make financial decisions that make sense and continue to make the HCO money while servicing the population the HCO cares for. Proposals for improvement must be attainable and within the HCO's capability to implement. People, facilities and equipment are needed to start a new branch of an HCO--which must be available for a new project to be approved. Some of the money can be designated for a specific area for future improvement. The HCO will watch the interest rates to determine the best time to put money back into the market and ensure they are paying the lowest rates possible.

## Pricing

Each healthcare organization (HCO) must determine how it wants to charge its customers. Some pricing is out of the HCO's control. For example, Medicare, Medicaid and some insurance companies define how they will pay the HCO, so if the HCO wants to accept these patients, it must accept the designated pricing. The HCO must determine if there is any flexibility within their set prices and when this flexibility should be exercised. The more flexibility within the type of payments accepted, the greater the chance of negative consequences developing for the HCO. For example, if the HCO chooses to accept patients represented by an insurance company which designates set payment for services, the HCO risks losing money on each service. It is nearly impossible to provide excellent care at cheap rates, but people want to pay low prices, so HCOs attempt to get customers by reducing prices. Doctors know their customers best and the skill required to service their customers, and should be involved in determining how much should be charged for services.

**Debt and equity**

It is important that a healthcare organization (HCO) makes sure that it balances the amount of money it borrows with the amount it brings in. If an HCO appears to, or actually owes a lot of money to many different organizations, it will have a problem getting money from a bank when needed. HCOs invest in facilities and equipment that increase in value over time. The amount of money that the investment increases by is known as equity. Equity can be borrowed against and used to get money to re-invest. It is important to use equity wisely because if it is used and cannot be repaid, the result is the loss of the very necessities for a HCO to remain in business. In order for an HCO to expand, it must have a plan in which it can see how it will pay off in the future the money it needs to start a new branch of the HCO.

**Multi corporate organizations**

Healthcare organizations (HCOs) are increasingly removing smaller branches and adding them and/or other businesses to the main HCO. If there is more than one healthcare facility in a city, they will often come together to form one large HCO, or join together but function as separate units. Healthcare facilities in several different locations servicing a variety of populations have come together to form large HCOs. These multi corporate HCOs combine assets, which gives them more of an opportunity to raise money for expansion. The forming of a large corporation or the acquisition of other businesses can be short-term and used to achieve a specific goal. The main HCO can give money to the smaller branch it buys to help better their investments. The HCO can buy a business offering a specific type of service for its benefit. For example, if an HCO needs someone to process lab tests, it can purchase a lab testing company with which it can negotiate a fair price, but also ensure that the lab test company is providing excellent service.

**HCO employees**

Because healthcare is a service-based industry, many people are employed by a healthcare organization (HCO). Some are independent contractors who work within the facility but are not on the payroll of the HCO. Some people work for the HCO who are not paid, called volunteers. Employees are necessary for an HCO to remain in business and their happiness makes an HCO run better. The HCO must be competitive in salary, benefits and working conditions, because each employee has a choice of employers. The employees and departments must effectively work together because most people visiting a healthcare facility will encounter more than one caregiver. Employees see and interact with the HCO's customers, so how they feel about the HCO and their jobs is important as they create an image of the HCO. An HCO provides a lot of jobs to the population it services, so employees need the HCO to be successful to maintain employment.

The Human Resources department creates a workforce plan which is used to determine how many people are needed to work in each department of the healthcare organization (HCO). Human Resources factors in how many people are employed and will continue to be employed for the period of time the workforce plan is created for. The salaries and other compensation for employees should be projected in the workforce plan. If there are known areas where salary or other benefits will change, these should be detailed in the workforce plan. Human Resources must communicate with the various department managers to get information required for the plan. As the organization changes, so should the plan and it therefore requires consistent evaluation. If the plan uncovers a need for new employees or a need for the retention of employees, Human Resources develops strategies to cover the needs. Human resource planning plays a critical role in the lives of employees. If there is a surplus of employees, the HCO may have to let some employees go.

It is better for a healthcare organization (HCO) to promote from within and invest money in making internal employees better. New employees are still needed and HCOs follow set protocols to bring these employees to the organization. The Human Resources department establishes how many employees are working for the HCO at a given time and how many employees are needed. Each occupation within the HCO has specific job duties, which are detailed in a job description which is used to make salary and requirements fair to all people working at the same job. How much the HCO will pay for a specific position is uniform and pre-determined based on the job. If there is any special treatment given to a certain type of applicant for recruiting purposes it is pre-determined and the tools used to bring new employees (including recruiting strategies) are detailed and uniform.

Pre-qualifications that are required of job applicants are pre-determined by the HCO. The HCO may require a degree or special training, for example, and if an applicant does not have these qualifications they will not be considered. Affirmative action policies are those which are mandated by the government and must me complied with. They often require a company to hire a certain number of minority employees. After the potential employees have been interviewed, the process for picking the people to be hired follows pre-set rules and must be in line with affirmative action. Once hired, employees should be put through consistent training regarding how the organization functions, benefits that will be received, and the goals of the organization. Most HCOs require new employees to work as conditional employees and will only become permanent after proving they can work successfully within the HCO.

**Training programs**

Employees are instrumental in the success of a healthcare organization (HCO). HCOs have responded by investing money into training employees because they are such important assets. HCOs offer new-hire training programs to ensure the employees are well informed of their benefits and the goals of the HCO. Most HCOs provide training to help an employee move up within the organization, including how to provide better customer service to patients. Loyal employees who work many years for the HCO will eventually retire and Human Resources provides training to help these employees make the transition. The HCO may even help those people who are laid off find other places of employment. If the HCO opens another branch or department, Human Resources will explain how these changes can make an impact on current employees, like the possibility of new jobs, for example.

**Salary and compensation**

Healthcare organizations (HCOs) employ many people and these people must be paid through salary and other compensation including benefits. Computer systems are used to manage the payment of employees because errors are detrimental to the HCO and the employee. Each job within the HCO is paid a predetermined amount based on the education and skills required for the job. Human resources maintain and update salary information. An HCO does not have an unlimited budget to pay for employees and sets limits on the number of employees working within the HCO through the use of position control. This is meant to assure there are only enough employees necessary to meet the needs and demands of the HCO. Some people within the HCO get paid per hour they work. Others get paid a salary which is a set figure that does not change even when more than 40 hours are worked. Both types of employee's wages are overseen by a payroll system which ensures each is paid correctly.

For a healthcare organization (HCO) to keep the best employees available, it must pay them based on how well they are performing their job functions. If employees are doing well, the HCO can respond by giving them extra money beyond their salary, called incentives. The amount an HCO can afford to pay employees, however, has to be in line with the company's profits. If the HCO is not doing well financially, it cannot afford to pay employees more. The HCO should evaluate employees fairly when determining who to give more compensation to. It is sometimes hard to determine what role each person within the HCO has played in the HCO's success. The HCO should make it clear to employees that an incentive is a bonus and may not happen again. Typically, upper management receives incentives first and the leftover is distributed to lower level employees.

Human Resources are responsible for the oversight of employee benefits. Every employee is required to pay certain taxes, and the payroll department automatically removes the amount from the employee's paycheck and pays the appropriate party including Social Security, Medicare, and federal and state taxes. The healthcare organization (HCO) is required by law to hold worker's compensation insurance coverage and unemployment insurance. Employers pay employees to take time off work for illness, specific holidays and some provide paid time off for personal or vacation time. Most HCOs offer health insurance coverage to their employees and automatically deduct the premiums from the employee's paycheck. The HCO also contributes money into the health insurance coverage reducing the cost for the employees. Some HCOs provide money for employees who work for the HCO for a certain number of years and retire—money which employees can receive in a lump sum or monthly.

### Employee evaluations

Employees of a healthcare organization (HCO) are subject to reviews, usually at least once a year, based on how well they are doing their jobs. The reviews are meant to determine areas where an employee is functioning well and areas where the employee may need additional training to become more in line with the HCO's goals. Measuring competency is one way to achieve a performance review, but is typically reserved for supervisors and professionals. Competency describes traits a person has that help him or her do her jobs, which can be analyzed objectively. To ensure the employees are happy working in the HCO, Human Resources gives regular questionnaires. The questionnaires can include questions about the employee's supervisors and about the HCO as a whole. It is important for the employees to know that they can answer the questions truthfully, and without fear of retribution, so they are not required to put their name or other identifying information on the survey. Human resources can determine areas where dissatisfaction lies and takes steps to make those areas better.

**Safety, discrimination and sexual harassment**

Healthcare organizations (HCOs) must maintain a safe working environment because they are regulated by the government to do so, and because of the nature of their business. Human Resources perform the specific job duty of ensuring safety regulations are met as set forth by the Occupational Health and Safety Act. Human Resources must also ensure that people are treated equally within the organization following the Family Medical Leave Act and the Civil Rights Act of 1964. To avoid issues of discrimination, many HCOs will look at the population they serve and determine the percentage of minorities and women who live in the population. The HCO then tries to match the percentages of employees they maintain with the general population. It is also important that the HCO addresses and trains employees to avoid sexual harassment issues. People have various opinions on what is actually considered sexual harassment, so the HCO should have a clearly stated policy on the issue.

**Grievance process**

Sometimes an employee has an issue or problem that they feel should be escalated because they are unhappy with the response they are given. Many healthcare organizations have an ombudsman office that Human Resources can refer the employee to. A representative from the ombudsman office will act as an intermediary to represent the employee in front of the necessary parties. The goal is to diffuse the situation. If this is not possible, and the employee is represented by a union, he or she can file a formal grievance which can result in the union bringing legal action against the HCO. Managers should know how to handle the grievance process to avoid the escalation to a lawsuit. Supervisors should keep a well-written account of the problem and look into the problem fairly. Human Resources should try to come up with compromise when available. Even if the employee is not represented by a union, his or her problems matter and Human Resources should take all complaints seriously.

### Service excellence programs

Many healthcare organizations (HCOs) implement service excellence programs to create a successful workforce. The theory behind these programs is that if employees are given the tools and encouragement to do their jobs at the highest quality possible, the employees will respond by providing superior performance. The HCO must provide leadership that cultivates a culture of excellence. The supervisors must recognize a good job and respond with praise so the employees know they are being recognized. Education programs are integral to the development of employees. The only way an employee can perform well is to know how to do his or her job. Employees can then expand on the minimum requirements to perform beyond minimal expectations. Training should also include customer service strategies and strategies to maintain a positive and happy attitude even in the midst of stressful situations. Customer contact is a huge part of an HCO employee's job, so it is important the employee knows how to convey a positive attitude even in the most difficult times.

### Transformational management

Many healthcare organizations (HCOs) encourage the use of transformational management. The goal of this type of management is to help employees get better through training and encouragement, rather than through discipline and reprimand. HCOs should train supervisors on strategies that will help them implement transformational management strategies. Many managers are trained to use punitive measures to get what they want from employees, so the transformational style may be new. Management should be well versed in the HCO's principles so they can communicate those principles effectively and clearly to the employees. Management is responsible for looking at their department and finding areas that are in need of improvement. Oftentimes, these improvements require money from the established budget. Sometimes the money from the current budget is used, so managers must look for areas that can be improved in the future to avoid their being ignored in the future budget.

### Human Resources

The Human Resources department of a healthcare organization is typically large and extensive. A chief operating officer leads Human Resources as a whole and underneath him or her is a vice president. Because Human Resources are responsible for so many different functions, it is branched into many different departments. One department is responsible for finding and bringing in new employees. Another is responsible for any income that employees receive in the form of money or benefits. Another department is responsible for ensuring each employee has the proper training for his or her job function. If the HCO offers any other plans that benefit employees that are outside of the heading of compensation, another department is created to oversee these programs. The Human Resource department is responsible for improvement in its quality and there is a separate department led by a supervisor who is responsible for overseeing the administrative and goal-oriented focuses.

**Plant system**

Healthcare organizations are large and must have space available for the many units contained in their facility. The healthcare buildings must be cleaned and maintained. The food service areas and waiting rooms must be maintained. The facility maintenance of an HCO is known as a plant system. Part of the responsibility of leadership of the plant system is to use the space within the HCO in the best way possible to provide safety, convenience and aesthetic appeal. When people visiting the healthcare facility feel secure and comfortable, they get better faster. If the HCO looks better, more people will want to visit, so putting money into the design aspects of the HCO is worthwhile. Medical equipment is necessary in an HCO so the design of the HCO must reflect the placement of these necessary items. Some departments of the HCO require more room, which must be provided for in the design of the HCO.

Plant services operate under a hierarchy created to oversee the departments. The department is led by a chief operating officer and below him or her is the vice president. One unit of plant services involves the building and equipment upkeep and improvement. Another department oversees the accrual and space necessary for new and existing materials. Another main department is responsible for the oversight of space used within the healthcare facility. One branch of this department is to ensure that the needs of people visiting the HCO are met. This includes hiring people to ensure the HCO is safe, providing shuttle service from the parking lot and greeting visitors upon arrival. The other branch oversees the upkeep of the facility, including cleaning the inside and maintaining the landscape outside of the facility.

The plant services department is evaluated to ensure it is meeting the standards set forth by the healthcare organization (HCO). One area that is evaluated is how well the plant services department completes all tasks requested of them. If their performance does not meet the needs of the HCO, the department is failing. Another area that is measured is how well the department uses money allocated in the budget. The department is responsible for investigating outside companies to find the best products at the lowest prices. The plant services department is evaluated on how well it retains its employees. Because the department is responsible for the aesthetic appeal of the organization, which is directly related to customer satisfaction, the department is evaluated on the how well they provide the upkeep of facility.

**Expanding or purchasing HCOs**

As healthcare organizations (HCOs) grow, they may decide to make a pre-existing healthcare facility better through remodeling and expansion. The HCO may choose to buy or rent a different facility or part of a facility. Either way, the HCO does not keep on its regular payroll a construction team to complete the work and must therefore hire people from outside of the organization. The HCO will generally ask for bids on a project to determine the best choice in who will complete the work. The National Fire Protection Organization created the Life Safety Code and is just one of many organizations whose regulations must be followed. It is important that the HCO choose a construction team that knows the regulations and will follow them. Money and resources may be needed to get the building in line with set guidelines and the construction team should make the HCO aware of any extra investment that will be needed as soon as possible.

**Catastrophic events**

Healthcare organizations (HCOs) must have a plan to handle a mass amount of people visiting the HCO at one time. In the event of any catastrophic event, either naturally caused or unnaturally caused, many people at one time may be in need of emergency medical care. In the event there is a need for a large amount of medical attention at once, the healthcare staff should stop any work they are doing that is not critical and attend to the large amount of incoming patients. There should be a team who can decipher the patients' symptoms and determine which area of the hospital a patient must be seen by. A team should look for places for the victims to stay in case they have lost their homes. Another group should be responsible for providing treatment to people who are in the hospital because of unrelated injuries. The HCO should have vendors in mind for any extra equipment or supplies that may be needed to meet the increased demand.

## Internal consulting groups

A successful healthcare organization (HCO) constantly evaluates its various parts to look for areas that can be improved. Many hire internal consulting groups that may oversee specific departments, or move around and analyze many departments for possible areas of improvement. The role of these groups is to perform 6 basic functions for the HCO. One role is to analyze the marketplace where the HCO exists. The group should constantly watch for alterations in the types of people living in the community the HCO services, or anything else that may need to be addressed by the HCO's upper management. Another role of consulting groups is to ensure the HCO they represent is in the best possible place for future growth. This means making sure the HCO's goals are consistently updated to reflect strategies that move the HCO forward. Another role of the groups is to make plans into the future that will meet the new goals. Another role is to look at other HCOs in the service area and look for any opportunities to capitalize on their successes and failures. The updating of medical equipment should be investigated to determine if the acquisition is cost effective. Many HCOs will work closely with people tied to government and a role of internal consultants is to foster these relationships.

## Areas of planning

There are many areas that must be considered when a planning unit evaluates the status of the population that the healthcare organization (HCO) services. The people within the community the HCO services must be analyzed to determine what types of illnesses have historically and may in the future affect them. Another area of examination is how the people of the service population feel about and react to healthcare services. Some market areas are poor and have little access to healthcare other than through government assistance. Other areas have high employment rates and high access to health insurance. This must be examined by the planning team so the HCO will know how and from whom it will be receiving payment. It is important for the planning team to determine how happy and how educated its employees are. The planning team should determine how many doctors are available to the population it services and what types of services they provide, to avoid over saturating the market with one type of physician.

## Consultants

Consultants, whether internal or external, should be used strategically. The task that is given to the consultants should be well defined and stated so there is little room for misunderstanding. The more information the consultant has about the area of concern, the better job he or she can do in fixing the problem. If the problem can be fixed by people already employed by the healthcare organization, it should be. Consultants who are experts about the specific problem should be used and if an expert cannot be found, gaining a second or third opinion is a good strategy. The consultants should not be left to work at their own pace and discretion. The HCO should maintain oversight and make sure the consultants are meeting expectations. There should be clearly defined avenues of communication for the consultants so they can work quickly and efficiently.

If the healthcare organization does not have the human resources available to employ internal consulting groups, it may choose to hire an outside company for certain functions. Outside companies can be used to evaluate the marketplace, investigate other healthcare organizations, determine and suggest areas where the HCO can improve and facilitate discussion within the HCO. One benefit of using an outside agency is that they are unaware of existing policies and practices and can give an unbiased viewpoint. Outside agencies have no vested interest in any one opinion and therefore can be a successful intermediary for more than one vantage point. The HCO can pick an agency that specifically handles a specific business problem to take advantage of their expertise. Outside agencies can be hired on for a set project and released so they do not remain on the HCO's payroll for an extended period of time.

## Marketing

Marketing in a healthcare organization (HCO) goes beyond simply bringing in patients to the organization. The marketing plan must consider how important the quality of the healthcare being provided is to the people needing it. The HCO must ensure it has doctors available to the patients brought in through the marketing plan and that it has the materials available to service those patients. Because there is typically an insurance company or some other party paying for the medical services provided, the HCO must factor in their marketing strategy the needs and wants of the companies actually paying. Some of the HCO's customers, whether they are patients or insurance companies, may feel that different healthcare services are acceptable in fixing their condition. It is important the HCO considers the inconsistencies in emotions about acceptable healthcare in their marketing plan.

It is important that a healthcare organization (HCO) identifies and caters their marketing strategies to a well-defined customer base. The HCO can look at the whole market and place each person into defined groups--which is a process called market segmentation. Market segmentation is important because it ensures that people are getting an appropriate marketing message based upon their circumstance. For example, elderly care is specific to seniors and money spent on marketing these services to 25 year olds is money wasted. The market can be divided based on income and any other factors that will have an effect on the customer's buying decisions. Once the market is segmented, the HCO must determine the best way to reach the customers in each group through a marketing strategy. These strategies will change and must be adaptable as the market changes.

A healthcare organization (HCO) must employ various strategies to determine the needs and wants of its customers so it can develop a marketing strategy that reaches the appropriate people with an appropriate message. Formal surveys are used to question any group of people, from patients to employees, to uncover areas that they want changed or addressed. The HCO can use the information to develop their goals specifically for a group's preference. To gain more information, the HCO can gather small groups of people from a specific market group into a focus group. This provides an environment where the HCO can learn even more about the specific needs of a group of customers and how to most successfully meet their needs. The HCO can identify problem areas by maintaining monitors in the facility. Monitors can be comment cards for employees or customers to fill out or the requirement of written incident reports when anything goes awry within the HCO. Finally, the HCO will require its supervisors to keep their ears open when working within the HCO. They should be asking questions and listening to employees and customers, which is an activity that requires the supervisors to spend time out of their offices and in the daily activities of the HCO.

Part of a healthcare organization's marketing strategy includes branding. The HCO wants people in the population it services to associate its facility with positive feelings. One way an HCO can induce a positive public image is to reach out and communicate with the people it services. For example, an HCO can send a monthly letter with recipes that are healthy including the HCO's name, information and logo. The HCO has now reached many people who will associate the brand with a positive message. The HCO can sponsor activities that people will enjoy. A food drive with carnival games for children can send a message that the HCO cares for the community. The food drive in no way asks the community to use the HCO's facility, but places a good impression in the minds of those who participate. The HCO can use the news media to convey a message or can tie the HCO to fixing a problem that the media identifies. If, for example, the media is discussing tobacco use among teens, the HCO can provide information to help teens stop smoking so the HCO can be tied into the story in a positive way.

Once the market is identified and segmented, a healthcare organization (HCO) uses strategic functions to determine the best strategies to align the HCO with the market. The HCO may need to adjust its goals as detailed by the governing board to reflect the findings of the needs and wants of the employees, customers, and other companies who the HCO must market to. The HCO must create a strategic position to make sure it is reaching its customers in the most effective way so they will begin using or continue to use the HCO. The HCO must consider how new and advancing medical equipment will affect the market. The HCO must determine how much money it can spend to get more customers. Determining what strategies other HCOs, either new or existing, are employing should be investigated to determine their effect on the strategic planning.

**Nurse characteristics**

The roles of nurses in the healthcare industry are diverse, but overall nurses are meant to provide patients with extended quality care. The American Nurses Association (ANA) has set forth what type of characteristics nurses should possess, beginning with the fact that nurses are meant to develop interactions with patients that help the patient feel better emotionally and physically. People are different and will react differently to health problems and nurses should be able to respond appropriately. The nurse should be able to provide healthcare based on medical knowledge as well as the unique situation of each patient. The nurse should be able to use education and apply it in medical situations to figure out what is wrong with a patient and administer appropriate care. A nurse should be part of some type of continuous education program. The nurse should be an advocate for the population as a whole when it comes to medical care.

**Institutional and community nurses**

Nurses either work in institutional nursing, meaning they work for a corporation or institution or they work in community nursing, working for the needs of the population in their service area. Institutional nurses meet the demands of many different settings, including hospitals and long-term care facilities, so a wide range of skills are required of each different type of nurse. The nurses are often specialized in a particular type of care based on the institution they work for. For example, a nurse in a neo-natal intensive care unit must have a different skill set than one working in a nursing home. Nurses who work in community nursing require a knowledge base that will help the population in general, including teaching how to avoid illnesses and maintain a healthy lifestyle. Some will teach the elderly how to exercise, while some will teach students how to care for themselves. There are many opportunities in both institutional and community care for any person interested in the nursing field.

### Advanced practice nurses

Most nurses have a bachelor's degree, but they can earn a masters to become advance practice nurses (APNs) who can take leadership roles or specialize in a specific area of nursing. Nurse practitioners perform many of the functions of a doctor and can see patients full-time unless a specific problem arises in which the patient needs a physician's care. Babies can be born with the help of nurse midwives. Anesthetics can be administered by nurse anesthetists, a process that is covered by Medicare. Some nurses with advanced education become case managers. Case managers investigate a person's illness and treatment options to determine the least expensive way for the patient to receive quality care. Nurses can work in management of a healthcare organization. The nurse's on-the-job training and advanced education prepare him or her to meet the demands of nursing management.

### Job duties

The following is a list of job duties a nurse must perform:

1. The nurse must care for patients by using either his or her judgment or by following the direction of a doctor or other healthcare staff, a job duty known as delivery.
2. The nurse must follow protocols while administering patient care and use his or her knowledge to ensure protocols are followed as closely as possible, a job duty known as appropriateness.
3. The nurse has a responsibility to provide quality care so that the person receiving the care and his or her loved ones are happy with the service, a job duty known as amenities and marketing.

4. The nurse should be involved in making sure a patient receives care when needed and without having to wait excessively, a job duty known as scheduling and recording.
5. The nurse should ensure quality care is being provided according to the goals and values of the organization and if that it not happening, should fix problem areas, a job duty known as performance improvement.
6. The nurse should provide input on how many people and what supplies will be required, a job duty known as planning and budgeting.
7. The nurse will help bring in new nurses and be a positive force in the staff so nurses will want to remain, a job duty known as human resources.

**Dealing with family members**

In times of severe illnesses, the person a nurse is caring for has family members at his or her side through the process. Because the nurse has so much interaction with a patient, the nurse will often be questioned as to the direction of care a patient is receiving. Nurses should be effective communicators, easing the mind of family members when possible and providing quality care to the patient. The nurse has to be able to educate the family about the specifics of an illness, tell the family or patients what administrative tasks must be completed, and give details about future care, which is all known as cognitive support. A nurse must also have the ability to perform emotional support to a family. The nurse needs to communicate with the person or persons who will be providing the most support for the patient and should be able to look at a family and find this person, or persons. The nurse should anticipate and respond to the needs of the family. Protocols are created to help a nurse provide emotional support.

**Patient care plan**

Nurses create unique patient care plans which respond to the needs and symptoms of the individual patient while following set protocols whenever possible. Sometimes a patient's illness cannot be treated based solely on a protocol and the nurse must adapt the protocol in those cases. The nurse must assess the patient based on medical history and by listening to input from the people caring for the patient. Most patients are not cared for by just one doctor, so the nurse should communicate with all of the patient's doctors to determine the best course of treatment for the patent. The care plan needs to include communication with the patient's family on what circumstances the patient will be faced with after leaving the hospital and take into account any special needs. The nurse should also evaluate the financial status and needs of the patient and how treatment will affect the patient's finances. The patient care plan should have a discharge plan which details when the patient will leave the healthcare facility.

**Nursing staff**

Because there is such an extensive number of nurses working for a healthcare organization who are specialized in many different areas, the nursing staff must be coordinated and overseen. A chief nursing officer (CNO) is generally responsible for the oversight of the nursing staff. His or her duties include ensuring the nurses have appropriate education, bringing in and keeping employees, and determining the job expectations of the nursing staff. Beneath the CNO are department managers called directors who oversee unit managers. The education requirements of nurses vary by profession. Professional certification rather than a bachelor's degree is sufficient in specific areas of nursing care while upper management is typically required to have education beyond a bachelor's degree. Registered nurses (RNs), for example, need a certification not a bachelor's degree to work in the field. Nurses who specialize in a field typically need a master's degree, which is a requirement of nurse practitioners.

Nurses have a variety of skill levels and many areas of nursing should be represented at any given time in a hospital. The nurses take part in determining how many and what type of nurses are necessary. The nursing budget includes the wages of the nurses employed, which is a flexible number. The variation of nurses working at a given time includes nurses in a managerial role who oversee people who are caregivers, but they are not nurses that can provide basic care. A table is used, which is typically on a computer program that requires input and will output the staffing needs of nurses for a given time frame. If there are a lot of people needing care or there are many with serious illnesses, staffing decisions must reflect the patients' needs. When using a staffing model, people with serious illnesses are designated a higher number than regular patients so the system will recognize the need for increased staffing.

**Scheduling system**

A computer program is generally used to analyze staffing needs and create a schedule. The program should be able to determine the right amount of nurses and other caregivers that will be required and also ensure the right type of nurses are working at all times. The systems should help managers make a difficult schedule so they do not have to waste human resources to complete the schedule. The system should be able to pick appropriate staff so that the organization does not have to pay for extra hours or to bring in nurses when there is a shortage. The system should create a month-long schedule that can be manipulated at any time if necessary. The system should recognize holidays and weekend shifts and spread the shifts out fairly. If an employee needs a day off, the system should make sure such requests are treated fairly among all employees.

**Nursing assignments**

The people in charge of assignments look at the nursing schedule and make manual adjustments based on needs of the hospital and problems with staff, including unforeseen circumstances like when personnel calls in sick. Nurses who are overworked because there are staffing problems are generally unhappy with their work environment. Part of a quality healthcare organization includes keeping employees happy, so staffing problems should be met with an increased staff whenever possible. If there is a need for more staff in one department that can be fulfilled by another department that has few patients, nurses can move over to cover the need. Many staffing systems can provide this service and can recognize the best placement of patients based on their medical needs and staffing available. If all else fails, there are groups of nurses who have the ability to work in many areas who can be called upon in a time of need. Nurses can be paid overtime or outside vendors who keep a nursing staff can be called upon. Any of those alternatives becomes an extra expense for the healthcare organization and the people being called in are often not as skilled as the normal nursing staff.

**Chains of communication**

Nurses have the most frequent and extensive contact with a patient. Nurses are essentially the eyes and ears for doctors within a healthcare organization. Nurses communicate with doctors to make sure that they have a plan of action for the patient that is detailed and complete. As the nurse monitors the activity of the patient, he or she is responsible for communicating his or her findings to the doctor. Nurses create patient care plans and monitor the patient and his or her family for any potential areas of concern that may need intervention. Nurses keep track of medication and care given to a patient. Nurses must remain in close contact with CSSs. Nurses must keep a written account or incident reports if any problem arises that could be questionable. Nurses communicate with families about the patient's illness and help the family in whatever way possible regarding the patient's medical condition.

## Nursing computer system

Information systems have been developed to evaluate the effectiveness of nurses and the care they provide. Patient-scheduling systems keep the schedules of patients and can therefore track problems or inadequacies in the treatment of patients in a timely manner. The expenses of a nursing unit are tracked through information technology, which can be used to find areas where costs can be reduced or eliminated. Because the staff schedule is kept on the computer, reports can be run to see who is or is not coming to wire and when more nurses were needed but were unavailable. The system can track how the nurses are servicing patients of various needs based upon the information nurses input into the system like patient care plans, for example. The system can track how long it takes nurses to care for a patient thus tracking nurses' productivity.

Information systems created to evaluate the effectiveness of nursing care record the illnesses patients are faced with, so the end result of the care given by nurses can also be tracked, including times when an error is made. When something goes wrong with a patient's care, the problem is recorded and input into the computer system so these deviations from quality care can be evaluated for improvements. The computer system can tell if a variety of nurses are available at a given time to provide quality care or if other structural standards are being fulfilled. The computer system can create surveys and the results of the surveys can be input so management can run reports and determine areas where customer service is lacking and can be improved. Doctors are also questioned to determine how happy they are with the nursing staff, to uncover any areas of concern or needs for improvement.

## Clinical support services

Diagnosis and treatment of illness is not the only demand patients have in the healthcare industry. Clinical support services (CSSs) cover helping patients with after care and doctors will establish the use of clinical support services when needed by the patient. A physician, for example, typically does not have the training to help a patient stop drinking alcohol, but can treat the damage to a patient's liver caused by extensive alcohol use. A doctor, after treating the patient's liver, can recommend CSSs to help the patient overcome his or her addiction. Laboratories that process test results are also CSSs. Healthcare organizations (HCOs) can chose to train staff in house to perform some of the job duties of a CSS, or can chose to pay a

CSS when necessary. A cost-benefit analysis of using a CSS must be completed by the HCO to ensure whatever path they chose ultimately best services patients' needs.

It is not cost effective for a healthcare organization (HCO) to outsource all of the necessary clinical support services (CSSs), because many departments within the HCO can provide the services. CSSs are still necessary for any services that are too difficult for in-house completion. If proper execution of a CSS can be completed in house, it should be, because that is a cheaper alternative than paying a CSS. If a physician has no ties to any particular CSS, they are not supposed to refer a patient to one CSS over another. Because of this, CSS providers must market to patients and physicians when the CSS can offer discounts for use. Insurance companies tend to pay in bulk for CSSs. These contracts are important to the CSS so they must offer excellent service at fair and competitive price. This may mean charging less for services to get an overall large contract.

### Training requirements

For clinical support services (CSSs) to be effective, they must be evaluated and measured for quality. A major area of quality for CSSs is technical quality. If sloppy work is completed or the employees are insufficiently trained to do their job correctly, technical quality is not achieved. A CSS expert should be well trained and have a formal education to backup their training. CSS experts require high salaries so they are typically placed in managerial roles over people with an informal education. The CSS experts should attend ongoing training, which should include tools to overcome professional disagreements between experts that sometimes arise. The CSS experts should also receive special training on how to oversee the nonprofessional staff working beneath them. Protocols are created for CSSs to follow. When the CSS experts and the nonprofessionals receive adequate training regarding accepted protocols, both can provide higher quality healthcare.

### Monitoring technical quality

How well clinical support service (CSS) specialists complete their job is analyzed and reviewed to find opportunities for increased quality. Quality can be traced by evaluating how well protocols are followed. The normal functions completed by CSSs should be monitored by people outside of the clinical support team, to look for areas of opportunity. The type of CSS that is provided to each patient is tracked in the patient record and these records can be a source to determine any areas where quality was unfulfilled. Mistakes and duplicate work can be tracked--which are both causes of technical quality failure. Tracking of end results compared to what the result should be to determine areas of mismatch is completed to ensure quality. The point of tracking quality should be to ensure a patient is receiving good treatment. Sometimes, duplicate work is required to fulfill a patient's needs. The point of finding mistakes is not necessarily to punish someone, but to stop the mistake from happening in the future.

**Discontinuing clinical support services**

A doctor may decide that a clinical support service (CSS) is appropriate and will ultimately help the patient, but a doctor cannot force a patient to use the CSS. Many factors can stop a patient from choosing a CSS. If the CSS is providing poor technical quality, the physician and patient may decide that using the CSS is too expensive or not worth the effort. CSSs become expensive when mistakes are made in testing or reporting results and if the CSSs are too expensive, the patient may refrain from using them. If the patient is unhappy with the service they receive from the doctor or the CSS they may ignore the doctor's advice and not use the CSSs. If a doctor or patient is unaware that a CSS is available, they will not take advantage of the service. Therefore, the CSSs must advertise their services.

**Needs of CSSs**

Each healthcare organization (HCO) must determine if it is cost effective to offer or use clinical support services (CSSs). The people who administer CSSs are often asked for input as to the future need and new areas of need for CSSs. Two models are used to determine the need of a CSS. One model multiplies the number of people who may need a CSS by the number of times that the use of a CSS has been needed, which is then multiplied by the number of times the CSS was actually used, which is then multiplied by how much of the market the specific HCO has. This equation, once completed, gives the amount of a particular CSS that is needed. The information input in the first model is non-specific, but is based on averages. The second model uses numbers from previous years of how many times a CSS was used and then uses forecasts to determine the future needs of CSSs.

**Competition**

The field of clinical support services (CSSs) is highly competitive and in order to remain in business, a CSS must process as much work as possible. Many healthcare organizations and physicians' offices have in-house CSSs that take up part of the market share. To remain competitive, a CSS must provide excellent service and most have patients fill out questionnaires to determine how happy they are with the service they have received. The CSS has to advertise as mush as possible to get doctors to use their services but, if patients are treated poorly when using the CSS, there are plenty of other CSSs the physician or patient can choose the next time around. Many CSSs who process tests for patients go to the physician's facilities to retrieve the tests rather than having a patient drive to the CSSs office. Members of a CSS team should be positive and pleasant to do business with, especially because it is such a highly competitive environment.

### Physician benefits

Many CSSs will give benefits to doctors, or physician amenities, if a doctor uses their service. This is an attempt to ensure the physician either begins using, or continues to use a particular CSS. The goal is to keep the physician happy. The CSS can offer a wide range of options they can perform for the doctor and get the physician results of any completed services quickly. The physician will want to keep their patients happy as they too rely on return customers, so a CSS willing to work with the physician to make patients happy is highly regarded. The CSS can offer software that will allow the doctor to input information the CSS can receive immediately making for faster service times in both receiving and sending information. Insurance can be verified and tests can be requested quickly and easily with the use of a computer system.

### Scheduling

CSSs must be fast, which requires a proper amount of staffing to meet customer demands. This can be a difficult process because, although some demand is normal, many medical conditions exist without forewarning and it is impossible to know beforehand what the demand will be. When a CSS provider receives a service request it is labeled emergency, urgent or schedulable. Emergency request must have immediate attention even if some quality issues are overlooked. Urgent requests are expected to be processed quickly, but also correctly. Schedulable requests can be satisfied at a set time that both the CSS and patient agree upon. The type of service a physician or hospital provides determines the type of demands they typically request. Emergency rooms will frequently have emergency demands for example. Computerized scheduling systems can be used to assess various factors and help design a schedule that will meet CSS's demands.

## Continuous improvement strategies

Clinical support services (CSSs) are analyzed to determine areas that can be altered for better quality. By consistently evaluating processes and comparing processes to other CSS providers, areas of need can be uncovered. If an area in need of improvement is discovered, the CSS provider can update protocols to reflect better ways of doing things. CSSs are impacted by medical advancements and the creation of technology that will enhance the CSS provider's quality. Any new processes the CSS provider accepts, is in the name of providing better quality help in customer satisfaction, which is important to any CSS provider. A good CSS provider will make the constant review of processes part of the standard activity. Employees will in turn seek areas in need of improvement and offer their insight into making the CSS's processes better.

## CSS budgeting

Clinical support service (CSS) budgets are important to the performance of the CSS. The CSS must have enough money to meet goals and expectations and to stay in business. The budget must allow the CSS enough resources to remain worthwhile to all of its customers. If another CSS can offer a better or more cost-effective alternative, the CSS will become unnecessary to the marketplace. The CSS must meet performance goals and make money for whoever is financially supporting the CSS. How well the CSS has performed in the past is a factor to be considered in the budgeting process. The budget must consider any quality initiatives set forth from CSS evaluation and must take into account any other issues that will potentially affect the CSS in the budgeted year or years. Diagnostic radiology is affected by work that must be redone, work that is done incorrectly, and work that takes too long to complete, which affects the budget and must be addressed. A pharmacy is concerned with better ways to track their supplies, using the least expensive drugs possible and problems with prescriptions from doctors all of which must be addressed and do affect the budget.

Managers of CSSs are responsible for assessing the cost associated with increased quality measures, protocols that are created and money needed for capital. The budget manager determines the future need for the CSS based on market share and the CSS manager must consider these forecasts in the budget. The budget manager looks at the past budget to see areas where the budget was met. The budget manager collects data to see how well the CSS is performing compared to other CSSs so goals can be set. The budget manager provides information regarding the assessment of finances provided by the finance committee of the board. Salary changes and increased cost of medical equipment are gathered by the budget manager. Line supervisors review the budget and make sure it is in line with maintaining customers' happiness. The line supervisor knows what affects the daily activity of a CSS so he or she should be the voice in ensuring the CSS is bettered by the new budget. Line supervisors represent all units of the CSS and should try and represent each unit equally during the budget process.

### New equipment or technology

Because the healthcare field is constantly developing new and better ways of providing medical services, new and better technology is also consistently designed. Clinical support service (CSS) managers look for these advancements and create programmatic proposals that reflect the CSS's need for different technology. It is important to understand that all technology is not necessary just because it is better. If the price of the new technology is more expensive than its potential benefits, it should not be purchased. A formula to determine how much the technology is worth has been created. The number of people who will need a service is multiplied by how much the new technology will help make the service better, which is multiplied by the dollar amount applied to the benefit of the service, which gives the total amount in dollars that buying new equipment will help the CSS for a year.

### CSS employees

Clinical support services (CSSs) cannot function without employees and they are responsible for finding and educating new employees on the specific job functions expected. Because customer service is such an important aspect of the CSS, it must be part of the training program. Education does not stop after new hire training. CSSs must keep updated credentials, which often require further schoolwork. Current employees who can be educated in more than one field are valuable assets to the CSS because they can fill multiple roles within the organization. Part of cultivating a positive work environment goes beyond paying employees a high salary. Employees need to know that their managers recognize good job performance and good managers will make positive employee feedback part of their overall management strategy. Financial incentives should be used in conjunction with feedback, and managers should avoid using one form of incentive but not the other.

People working for clinical support services (CSSs) need to feel like they have a secure and long-term employment and if they do not believe that, they may look for a company who can provide it. The number of customers a CSS services drives the amount of employees who are needed. When the amount of customers using clinical support services increases or declines there must be a change in the number of employees. A CSS can meet the change by finding better practices so employees can do their job faster. The people working for the CSS who are not full-time, permanent employees can be increased or reduced to meet the need of the CSS. The CSS can lay off workers or allow them to work extra hours to meet a changing demand for service. Firing current employees or brining on new employees will adjust the number of employees. Temporary companies can be contacted to meet a temporary demand.

**CSS management**

A clinical support service (CSS) manager must be well trained and knowledgeable in the medical industry. The career is demanding and the responsibilities are numerous. Not only must the CSS manager have technical knowledge, but he or she must know how to manage people as well. Most CSSs have a manager who is a doctor and one who is not, so both parts of the equation are covered. Under an umbrella of a CSS, there may be many sites offering a variety of services. All must communicate and meet the demands of the CSS while working as individual units. The main CSS must communicate its value statement, provide employees and supplies, provide a manager to each unit of the CSS, help when disputes arise and make necessary changes to foster success. Many smaller units can report to the management of a larger unit; which, therefore, requires fewer managers for the CSS to pay and train.

CSS managers who are doctors and employed by a healthcare organization (HCO) are known as hospital-based specialists and can be paid differently based on an arrangement made between the doctor and HCO. If the doctor signs a contract with the HCO, he or she earns a paycheck continuously and is offered other incentives that the HCO offers all employees. The contract is very specific as to what exactly the physician will be responsible for, which gives the doctor the freedom to earn money separately for services not detailed in the contract. Rather than being an employee of the HCO, the doctor can remain self-employed and be paid per service he or she performs. The doctor can pay the HCO to work in their facility through a rental arrangement. Some independent doctors will pay part of their profits to the hospital in return for using their facility. Professional managers who are not physicians have the same type of salary arrangements as doctors, but are typically working full-time for the HCO.

### Patient results and work completion

Most clinical support services (CSSs) determine how well they are doing by studying the end result of patient care. If a CSS is involved in an end result that is either unexpected or could be avoided, the problem is addressed to improve future performance. Test results that determine an illness do not change the end result for the patient, unless done incorrectly, so the way the test is performed should be evaluated. The methods which clinical support service representatives employ to complete their work are evaluated for efficiency. The following of protocols and determining if specific tests are done correctly can both be monitored to determine how well an employee is doing his or her job. Many CSS managers will establish routine tests to determine if their CSS is in compliance with quality results. The tests are performed frequently enough to see a pattern for each individual or CSS being tested.

### Customer and doctor satisfaction

Surveys and questionnaires are used to determine how happy a customer of a clinical support service (CSS) is with the service they have received. Another way to ensure quality service is being provided is to hire people to randomly do business with a CSS while secretly recording their experience. The CSS can also ask normal patients to meet and discuss their experience with the CSS. Because a CSS relies on doctors sending patients to use their services, it is important for the CSS to determine how happy the doctors are with the service of the CSS. The CSS can determine this by asking the doctors to fill out a questionnaire once a year. Gathering patient and doctor responses is not enough to improve a CSS. The CSS must act on the information. The CSS can do this by a variety of methods, including providing more training for its staff or increasing its budget to make way for new technology or more employees.

### Palliative care

Some patients have received all of the medical treatment available and are still going to die because of an illness, but still need care called end-of-life (EOL) care; EOL care can be either palliative or hospice care. Palliative care is provided when there is no way to make a patient better physically. Instead, healthcare specialists can be supportive emotionally and reduce the physical suffering of the patient through the use of medication. Because some people with life-ending illnesses are in a healthcare facility, while others are in their homes, palliative care is available for both. Hospice care is available for those people with imminent life-threatening illnesses that cannot be cured. Once the patient is no longer receiving medical attention to alleviate a disease, Medicare and most insurance companies will pay for hospice care. Many untrained people who want to give their time to help ill people are part of hospice care programs. The goal is to make the patients happy and at ease during the last moments of their lives.

**Nursing homes**

The most commonly used long-term care facility is a nursing home. Nursing homes provide care for people with a wide range of illnesses and diseases. Some are there to care for elderly patients while some have staff that helps people overcome an illness or injury. Most nursing homes are owned by corporations which make money from the facility. Some are owned by businesses not trying to make money or by other types of individuals or groups who own the nursing home to serve a community and not to make money. Some are government owned. Nursing homes have had some recent trouble staying afloat financially because they are not being used enough. People are requiring specific types of services that many nursing homes cannot provide to everyone. The American Healthcare Care Association (AHCA) monitors nursing home quality and there are many complaints that have been found valid by the AHCA.

Certified nursing assistants (CNAs) make up the biggest portion of the caregivers at a nursing home. There is not a lot of education required to be a CNA and they are not paid well. It is, however, a difficult job because CNAs provide the most basic care for patients, including helping them in the bathroom and lifting them into wheelchairs. Good nursing home management will recognize the plight of CNAs and help them whenever possible, especially in the area of education. Medicare and Medicaid pay the highest percentage of nursing home fees. Insurance companies and the people or families of the people in the nursing home pay the rest. Medicare and Medicaid do not have the deepest pockets and pay nursing homes based on a state's population. Medicare simply does not pay enough to cover the entire nursing home expense and patients suffer from nursing homes that do not have the best supplies or staff.

## Nursing home alternatives

Most people late in life would rather live in their own homes rather than move into a nursing home or other long-term care facility. A good alternative is to provide housing where people can live independently but still have close access to healthcare providers in times of need. Unfortunately, there are too few of these types of facilities and they are often too expensive for most elderly people. People who want to stay in their homes should be assisted by healthcare organizations with care services that can be delivered at their home. If they cannot afford to pay out of pocket for these services or do not have insurance to cover the expenses, home owners can use the equity in their homes to pay for the services. The elderly person may need to change his or her house to accommodate a need, such as the need of a stroke patient to be in a wheelchair. The government will help the elderly pay for housing when in financial need.

# Practice Test

## Practice Questions

1. What type of software is used in the healthcare industry to evaluate costs and track patient care?
   a. Statistical software
   b. Spreadsheets
   c. Database management software
   d. Simulation software

2. When a healthcare provider visits patients away from the office, how can that provider access the patient's medical records?
   a. Electronic data interchange
   b. A terminal-host system
   c. A client-server system
   d. Mobile computing

3. What is the largest concern that healthcare management must deal with as more providers and patients use the internet to access healthcare information?
   a. Privacy
   b. Usage
   c. Email communications
   d. Web page development

4. How can a healthcare organization reduce data redundancy and maintain data consistency?
   a. By limiting access to information
   b. By controlling access to networked computers
   c. Through the use of databases
   d. By using encryption software

5. What type of database is most often used in the healthcare industry?
   a. Operational database
   b. Hierarchal database
   c. Analytical database
   d. Data warehouse

6. What is the most common way in which the healthcare industry protects private information?
   a. Public key encryption
   b. Virus protection
   c. Passwords
   d. Data backup and recovery

7. In what type of system are patient records maintained in the healthcare industry?
   a. Object-oriented databases
   b. Order-entry systems
   c. Results-reporting systems
   d. Clinical data repository

8. Which of the following is not a reason why a healthcare organization should develop strategies regarding the use of information technology?
   a. To ensure that the organization's standards are met
   b. To ensure that computer systems are used at optimum value
   c. To ensure that patient needs are met
   d. To determine the amount of money spent on computer systems

9. Which of the following terms describes the format information takes when entered into a computer system?
   a. Data warehouse
   b. Data dictionary
   c. Project organization
   d. Information system strategy

10. What is the primary advantage of using medical imaging systems and radiology information systems?
   a. The ability to view images
   b. The ability to track patient exams
   c. The ability to input patient symptoms
   d. The ability to make a diagnosis

11. Which type of information system helps healthcare providers diagnose and treat patient symptoms?
   a. Nursing information systems
   b. Laboratory information systems
   c. Clinical decision-support systems
   d. Medical imaging systems

12. What is the primary reason that healthcare organizations use financial information systems?
   a. Shareholder demands
   b. To improve patient care
   c. To create financial reports
   d. Government regulations

13. What is the purpose of executive information systems?
   a. Monitor the human resources of a healthcare organization
   b. Ensure proper functioning of a healthcare organization
   c. To minimize costs
   d. To make a profit

14. Which type of managed care system provides patients with healthcare services at a prearranged price?
   a. Preferred provider organization
   b. Exclusive provider arrangement
   c. Health cooperative organization
   d. Health maintenance organization

15. Which of the following is not a component of a decision-support system?
   a. User interface
   b. Model library
   c. Model editor
   d. Database management system

16. What are computer systems that hold private information called?
   a. Clinical systems
   b. Integrated systems
   c. Expert systems
   d. Consumer information systems

17. What method does the Health Insurance Portability and Accountability Act suggest as the most effective way of ensuring that a patient's personal information is not attached to their medical records?

a. Encrypting stored data
b. Password protecting computer systems
c. Limiting access to computer systems
d. Using a special code rather than a patient's name

18. Which of the following is a characteristic of a government hospital?

a. Not for profit
b. Research based
c. Earn a profit for the owner
d. None of the above

19. What is the main feature of a healthcare organization (HCO)?

a. Similar medical services are offered at a central location
b. Different medical services are offered at a central location
c. Different medical services are offered at various locations
d. Healthcare providers refer patients to other providers within a network

20. What type of organization ensures that financial transactions are completed fairly for both the insured and the company paying for benefits?

a. The Joint Commission on Accreditation of Healthcare Organizations
b. The American Osteopathic Association
c. A healthcare organization
d. A quality improvement organization

21. What system is used by healthcare organizations to determine the fees that should be paid per type of illness?

a. Insurance rating system
b. Healthcare provider information system
c. Prospective payment system
d. None of the above

22. What is the system used by healthcare organizations to ensure that customer service is monitored and improved?
   a. Strategic planning
   b. Continuous quality improvement
   c. Mission statement development
   d. Guidelines of expected behavior

23. Which organization creates standards for healthcare organizations that detail performance goals for managers and supervisors?
   a. Performance improvement teams
   b. Clinical systems
   c. The Plan Do Check Act
   d. The National Center for Healthcare Leadership

24. The governing board of a healthcare organization acts as a liaison between which groups of people?
   a. The contributors of the healthcare organization and insurance companies
   b. The healthcare organization and its contributors
   c. The healthcare organization and insurance companies
   d. The healthcare organization and regulatory organizations

25. Which individual is typically chosen to be the primary representative of the healthcare organization's board?
   a. The chairman of the board
   b. The board's legal counsel
   c. The chief financial officer
   d. The chief executive officer

26. Which of the following goals is not reflected on the operation balanced scorecard of a department within a healthcare organization?
   a. Demand for service
   b. Physical units
   c. Inputs
   d. Quality of care

27. What is the name of the separate governing board that oversees a healthcare center within a healthcare organization?
a. Subsidiary board
b. Strategic board
c. Financial board
d. Governing board

28. Which aspect of a healthcare organization detects areas within the organization that are not in compliance with expected results?
a. The executive committee
b. The cybernetic system
c. The information technology department
d. The standing committee

29. What is the purpose of an epidemiologic planning model?
a. To measure the population base of a geographic area
b. To measure epidemic illnesses in an area
c. To determine the types of doctors working in a specific area
d. To determine the number of people needing the services of an HCO

30. How do healthcare organizations maintain a chain of communication between departments and the governing board?
a. The mesh model
b. Information technology systems
c. The executive committee
d. None of the above

31. Which of the following is an example of a secondary prevention of illness?
a. A flu shot
b. Prescribing pain medication
c. Performing a biopsy
d. Immunizations

32. What is the purpose of applying a decision model when diagnosing a patient's illness?

a. To determine which medication to prescribe
b. To order the correct lab tests
c. To ensure that the physical and monetary price of a procedure is necessary for proper treatment
d. To determine a specialist for referring the patient

33. Which of the following terms describes the standards for what resources will be required in the completion of a medical procedure or patient care?

a. Continuous improvement
b. Clinical performance
c. Patient management protocols
d. Clinical expectations

34. How do healthcare organizations weigh the price of care for an illness against the expense of avoiding the illness?

a. By using a decision theory model
b. By establishing preventive healthcare strategies
c. By using financial analysis ratios
d. By using healthcare analysis software

35. What is the name of the system that evaluates doctors and ensures that physicians are qualified to provide medical care?

a. Accreditation
b. Licensing
c. Privileging
d. Board certification

36. How do healthcare organizations determine the number of physicians that are required to service the needs of the community where the organization is located?

a. By implementing a physician recruitment plan
b. By using a conceptual planning model
c. By using economic analysis
d. By performing demographic studies

37. What is the purpose of the Behavioral Risk Factor Surveillance Survey?
   a. To determine the health risks in a community
   b. To help healthcare organizations provide better services to the community
   c. To determine the types of people who will seek healthcare
   d. To help healthcare organizations become more competitive

38. What is the purpose of transaction accounting?
   a. To track payments received from insurance companies
   b. To determine the variable costs of a healthcare organization
   c. To track services provided to patients
   d. Locating and tracking financial dealings that have a bearing on the healthcare organization

39. Which of the following is detailed in the long range financial plan of a healthcare organization?
   a. Short term loans
   b. The monies earned and spent by the healthcare organization
   c. Expected future capital expenditures
   d. Future personnel needs

40. What is the main reason that healthcare organizations in different locations and that service different populations come together to form a larger healthcare organization?
   a. To increase the customer base
   b. To provide more services
   c. To combine assets and expand the business
   d. To increase the number of physicians on staff

41. Which of the following is not detailed in the workforce plan created by the human resources department of a healthcare organization?
   a. The number of people needed in each department
   b. The salaries and other compensation paid to employees
   c. Strategies for finding new employees
   d. The number of employees needed during the duration of the workforce plan

42. When an employee of a healthcare has an issue or problem that needs resolving, which office within a healthcare organization can act as an intermediary between the employee and the other party?

a. Human resources
b. The ombudsman office
c. The employee's union
d. The grievance department

43. What is the goal of transformational management?

a. To improve procedural processes
b. To facilitate a change in management
c. To use training and encouragement to improve employee performance
d. To help with the reorganization of a healthcare organization

44. Which of the following is not a responsibility of the leadership of the plant system of a healthcare organization?

a. To create a safe and comfortable environment
b. To provide efficient placement of medical equipment
c. To design an aesthetically pleasing atmosphere
d. To ensure that equipment operates correctly

45. What is the most important consideration when assigning tasks to a consultant?

a. Ensure that tasks are well defined
b. The experience of the consultant
c. Time constraints
d. The relationship between the consultant and the healthcare organization

46. Which type of marketing strategy helps a healthcare organization determine areas that are in need of change?

a. Focus groups
b. Direct observation
c. Comment cards
d. Formal surveys

47. According to the American Nurses Association (ANA), what is the most important characteristic that a nurse should possess?

a. Knowledge of healthcare procedures
b. Positive interaction with patients so that patients feel better emotionally and physically
c. Ability to understand the patient care instructions given by a doctor
d. Attention to detail and accuracy

48. What is the purpose of a patient care plan?

a. To address the needs and symptoms of a patient
b. To list medications and treatments needed by the patient
c. To help the patient's family care for the patient after discharge
d. To detail a patient's medical history

49. How can a healthcare organization ensure that there is adequate staff available to care for patients based on the patients' medical needs?

a. Allowing nurses to set schedules
b. Communication between doctors and nursing supervisors
c. Using patient-scheduling systems
d. Using staffing systems

50. What is the most important element for providing quality clinical support services?

a. Proper use of information technology systems
b. Proper training of clinical support services employees
c. Providing programs that meet the needs of the community
d. Accurate testing and reporting results

## Answers and Explanations

1. B: Spreadsheet software provides users with a way to manage and manipulate large sets of numbers. The healthcare industry uses spreadsheets to evaluate costs and track patient care. Statistical software is used to analyze input from the user by applying statistical methods to the data. Database-management software is software that allows the user to create access and manipulate a variety of databases, or collections of information. Users can compare information contained in databases. Simulation software creates an image of the information that needs to be analyzed so the user can experiment with the data without changing the original data.

2. D: Many times healthcare providers do not have access to a desktop computer when visiting patients away from the office. Mobile computing is a type of technology that can be used to access and manipulate data away from an internet connection. A laptop or other mobile device is used, but the information the user needs to access must be transferred to the mobile computer from the main computer before the information can be altered. Electronic data interchange, or EDI, is the term used to describe information sent back and forth between terminals without a person involved in the exchange. A terminal-host system is a centralized system that uses a main computer to process information and perform all computing tasks.

3. A: There are many concerns that management must deal with when the Internet is the main communication tool in an organization. Privacy is the most important concern and needs to be protected. Protection can include firewalls or putting information into code that hackers would not be able to decipher. Of lesser concern, internet usage within an organization must be monitored so employees do not access inappropriate websites or accidentally create security risks to the system. E-mail must be strictly monitored by management to ensure that personal e-mails are not being viewed, downloaded and forwarded. Email also puts the organization at risk for viruses. Management is responsible for ensuring that employees are using email appropriately and developing policies to ensure employees know their expectations. System administrators should be used to review web sites and authorize the creation of new web pages.

4. C: Databases are used to store information. Data redundancy is reduced and data inconsistency can be maintained and eliminated by the database. Databases fix most

of the problems related to data redundancy. This in turn strengthens the integrity of the data. Through the use of a database, different departments can access and see information stored on the database. Privacy is better maintained because one central database can be protected rather than multiple file sources.

5. B: The healthcare industry typically uses hierarchal databases for large amounts of complicated information and relational databases for information that is easily input into a spreadsheet type of application like employee information. Hierarchal and network models have specific lines to which the branches are connected to each other. Information has to be sent from the main department to its subsequent branches in a line formation. The structure of the databases makes it difficult to search the databases because they are not specifically named.

6. C: Privacy or confidentiality protection of databases is important in the healthcare industry because information in the databases is personal and most patients would not want their private information accessed by anyone outside of their healthcare providers. Management must protect individual records and the database in its entirety. Passwords are the most common way to limit numerous people from obtaining private information. Virus protection is necessary because people try to intentionally harm or completely ruin databases and operating systems. Networks and floppy disks are the main avenues through which viruses are passed so software should be installed to protect the system. Data backup and recovery systems ensure that information maintained in the healthcare computer system is saved and can be retrieved for later use.

7. D: The healthcare industry uses a clinical data repository (CDR) to maintain patient's records. These records include when they seek healthcare, their financial status with the medical facility, the conclusion of tests performed on the patient, and surgical procedures pertaining to the heart. Object-oriented databases make objects and text searchable. An object-oriented database management system (OODBMS) provides a fast way to access images and sound information and understands multiple programming languages. Order-entry and results-reporting software provides communication between departments when medical treatments are not performed in one office.

8. C: The four reasons why a healthcare organization should develop strategies regarding the use of information technology include the following: to ensure the information technology is best used to meet an organization's standards, to make sure the computer systems are being used at their optimum value, to manipulate the

computer systems technologically to meet the unique goals of the organization, and to determine how much money will be spent on the computer systems.

9. B: Part of the planning process for the use of an information technology system should include the format information will take when entered into the computer system. A data dictionary can be created which gives examples of and defines the format of data; when a user needs to enter information, the dictionary can be consulted. Information is exchanged between the departments of an organization and between medically-related businesses outside of the organization. This creates the need for use of the same type of data language, providing the systems with the ability to exchange information. Because this is an important issue for the healthcare industry as a whole, groups like the American National Standards Institute and the Health Industry Bar Code Supplier Labeling Standard have been formed to create common data formats.

10. A: Medical imaging systems and radiology information systems give doctors the ability to view images more extensively. Pictures can be taken and manipulated with medical imaging systems. Patient exams, including when they will occur and the outcome of the exam, are produced by radiology information systems. Radiology information systems can compile information for management needs. The computer has the ability to help doctors in the field of radiology by giving the doctors several possibilities when determining the best way to handle a patient's problems.

11. C: Discovering the cause of a patient's symptoms and the best way to relieve the patient's symptoms can be investigated by doctors through the use of clinical decision-support systems (CDSS). Passive CDSS systems organize the information in a functional and orderly fashion so the doctor can easily analyze the patient's information. In an active CDSS, known medical information is stored in the active CDSS so the computer can analyze patient's problems and apply known medical treatments to give the doctor some suggestions for how best to treat the patient. Nursing information systems help nurses determine the best patient care, oversee critical patients, and oversee groups of nurses. Laboratory automation is the process by which computers send and receive data from laboratory instruments.

12. D: Financial information systems are important to the healthcare industry because the industry is subject to government oversight and there are many providers offering the same type of services, which creates a competitive environment. Financial information systems have the ability to track costs and produce reports so management can make sound financial decisions. The financial

information systems consists of daily activity regarding finances and data from external sources (including government and market data), and strategic organization plans that are unique to the financial mission of each healthcare location.

13. B: The management of a healthcare organization must ensure every department is functioning properly and that the output of the organization is satisfactory to the owners of the organization. An executive information system (EIS) is designed to monitor how all areas of an organization are functioning and provides upper management a way to retrieve the data as a whole or in smaller pieces to be analyzed. Human resources information systems indicate how the employees are functioning, including the rate at which they are leaving the company or getting terminated, and the level of happiness they have with their jobs. Computerized resource utilization systems help minimize costs and ensure that resources are used accurately and efficiently. Scheduling systems are important because part of making a profit requires having healthcare providers with time to perform procedures and visit patients.

14. D: When a group of doctors or practices provide medical care to a set of defined people, the doctors are said to be involved in managed care. Health maintenance organizations (HMOs) are physicians that see patients within a specific insurance plan for a prearranged price set between the insurance company and HMO. A preferred provider organization (PPO) is a physician who provides medical services for a lower cost to a predefined group of people. If a person under a PPO insurance plan sees a doctor within the PPO network, the medical services will be charged by the PPO at a lower rate. Exclusive provider arrangements (EPAs) are developed when a company pays a specific physician to provide medical services to all of their employees without the use of an insurance company.

15. C: A decision-support system (DSS) contains the following elements: user interface, model manager, model library, database, database-management system, and a report writer. Data is input through the user interface. A model manager accesses information that has been created to evaluate a problem. The model library contains the various models used to analyze a problem including the use of math, visual displays, and financial models that determine possible outcomes. The DSS gets information from a database which is usually a relational database. The database management system oversees and guides the communication between the user and the database. The outcomes of using the DSS are provided to the user through the report writer.

16. A: Because computers in the healthcare industry contain personal and private information, they must be guarded through the use of information technology. The computer systems that hold private information are called clinical systems. The computerization of medical records with specific data on people using healthcare services has led to the need for increased security measures. Expert systems are a type of DSS system that can have authority over and make decisions about areas needing support in the healthcare field. The expert system has several parts including a section with known information, a section that holds information called a database and a section that applies rules to determine possible outcomes. Consumer information applications provide information about a doctor's experience, procedures performed, general health information, and healthcare trends.

17. D: Because the personal medical information of patients is contained in computer files, the Health Insurance Portability and Accountability Act (HIPAA) regulated the standard of protection required for patient information. Mandating the concealment of medical history will reduce the attempt of insurance companies to discriminate based on the information. Streamlining HIPAA processes across many different healthcare organizations requires HIPAA to define how each organization should comply. The Working Group for Electronic Data Interchange is a network of healthcare-related people who have formed to design policies for information management. A system must be created to use a special code rather than a name and social security number to label patients so personal information is not attached to their medical records.

18. B: The role of hospitals has evolved over time. They were first meant to provide medical services to groups of people in a central location. As technology has improved to meet the demands of medical practices, hospitals are needed to house technology so procedures can be performed that require longer term care than a physician's office can provide. Hospitals can be owned by the government, businesses that are paying for the hospital without making money and companies that are paying for the hospital to make money. Government hospitals are research based and partner with schools or are designed to meet some need within the general public. Government hospitals cannot be tied to a church. Some businesses buy hospitals, called not-for-profit hospitals, which are meant to help a community but are not meant to earn the owners money. Some groups of people or businesses purchase a hospital to make money and these are called for-profit hospitals.

19. B: Because government regulations reduced the amount of money medical providers could charge for services, coupled with the fact that the government could not afford to pay for people without insurance, medical providers have had to respond by creating strategies to make money. Medical providers do this by creating criterion to evaluate their services against goals called benchmarks and by weighing themselves against others providing similar services. Many banded together in a central location with other providers offering different medical services to create healthcare organizations (HCOs). Centrally locating physicians means they can share expenses and work together to create cost-saving strategies. HCOs are convenient to patients, acting as a one-stop shop for medical services. Some diversity exists in the success of HCOs because their success largely depends on variables such as the type of customers within the population they service and the HCO's location.

20. D: Companies who pay medical benefits on behalf of those in need use quality improvement organizations (QIOs) to ensure that the financial transactions are completed fairly for both the insured and the company paying for benefits. The Joint Commission on Accreditation of Healthcare Organizations (JCAHO) and the American Osteopathic Association are two agencies that ensure hospitals are following required guidelines. Their oversight is required by insurance companies and other people who financially fulfill patient's obligations. The government has similar agencies that ensure that financial transactions are completed within set guidelines. In order to make alterations or create a new hospital, the hospital must frequently obtain a certificate of need from the state government.

21. C: The prospective payment system (PPS) was designed to determine a fee that would be paid per sickness, referred to as a diagnosis related group (DRG) by Medicare for patients entering the hospital. Doctor's fees were determined by the relative value scale. Insurance companies followed suit and set limits on their payments. Because the various groups adopted the same strategy, HCOs had to accept the terms to remain competitive.

22. B: Because the healthcare organization (HCO) is dynamic, customer service must constantly be monitored and made better, which is a theory known as continuous quality improvement (CQI), created by W. Edwards Deming. How well the HCO is functioning and CQI must be analyzed by quantitative analysis and comparison to set standards or benchmarks. An HCO cannot be successful financially or in any other way without bringing in people to use its services. Developing strategies to maintain the people already using the medical provider and developing strategies to bring more people into the practice is another aspect of CQI. It is important that

those who work within the organization know they are valued and that their voice is heard.

23. D: The National Center for Healthcare Leadership creates standards for good managers. The performance of healthcare supervisors can be weighed against these standards. After reviewing the results of the supervisor's review, the HCO can design a personalized development plan, which is a plan of action to improve the supervisor in areas of need. Performance improvement teams (PITs) are formed to create new and better business tactics. Clinical systems need technical and logistic support from the HCO to function properly. This support includes detailed and up-to-date information on the people needing medical services. Plan Do Check Act (PDCA) or the Shewhart cycle is a system that helps PITs form new ideas and carry them out.

24. B: A group of people oversee the entire HCO and are called a governing board. Governing boards are necessary to ensure everyone contributing to the HCO is working together effectively so goals created by the board for the HCO are achieved. The governing board acts as a liaison between the HCO and everyone contributing to it. Without customers, or stakeholders, an HCO cannot function and it is up to the board to make sure both groups of people are happy. The overall purpose of board members is to make the most money possible for the owners of the HCO and they are measured by how much money they can make for the organization.

25. D: The people who are on the board of an HCO are typically temporary and the board job is not their primary source of employment. The board makes determinations together but their plans must be set into action by one person. A chief executive officer (CEO) is chosen by the board and the individual chosen is the main representative of the board. He or she leads the employees within the organization and is the contact point for those people interacting with the HCO outside of the organization. The CEO must be knowledgeable in every aspect of the HCO because he or she is the communication source between the board and the remainder of the HCO.

26. C: Departments within a healthcare organization (HCO) have goals they must meet and their performance is tracked in an operation balanced scorecard. One area on the scorecard reflects how much the HCO is being visited--known as demand for service. The number of clients a HCO is seeing and how that number has increased or decreased is a measurable area on the scorecard. Resources are a measurable area on the operation balanced scorecard. One part of the area of resources is

known as physical units. Management must project how many employees are needed at a given time, at what times equipment can be used, and how much inventory is on hand. The operation balanced scorecard has an area called "outputs" which is designed to evaluate the production of a healthcare organization (HCO). An important area to consider is how well the organization is supplying service to patients requesting care. The operation balanced scorecard has an area called "quality of care" which is meant to evaluate the level of care the healthcare organization (HCO) is providing.

27. A: A healthcare organization (HCO) often has many different healthcare centers under its umbrella. Each center can have a separate governing board, called a subsidiary board, that communicates with and report to each other and to the main HCO board. Subsidiary boards are important because they are located within the community they serve and therefore know their patients and their marketplace best. Because the healthcare centers under an HCO's umbrella can differ in services they provide, subsidiary boards ensure that people who are familiar with the specific types of services being offered are represented on the board. Having boards for separate organizations makes it easier if the separate healthcare organizations decide to become one in a joint venture because each HCO involved has a board representing its unique interests.

28. B: There are many departments within a healthcare organization. Management of the people working in each department is essential and a supervisor is assigned to each group to oversee activity, making it a cybernetic system. A cybernetic system is one that is overseen by either a human or computer to ensure it is functioning correctly. The supervisor of a healthcare organization (HCO) cybernetic system must detect areas that are not in compliance with expected results and make necessary changes to regain compliance. Standing committees, such as an executive committee, are often given responsibilities from the board. The standing committees should be given detailed tasks to complete and timelines for completion to ensure they are in fact performing the function they are assigned. If a standing committee is not specialized in a certain area that must be addressed, the board can form an ad hoc committee for a designated timeframe. The ad hoc committee is tasked with investigating a problem and finding solutions for the governing board.

29. D: The governing board must assess the need for growth of their healthcare organization (HCO). In order to determine how many people within the population surrounding an HCO will need to use its facilities for inpatient or outpatient care, an epidemiologic planning model is used. The model is used to determine what types of

doctors will be needed based on past use. The model divides the actual usage of a hospital for either a particular procedure or number of customers in the previous year by the total number of the particular procedure or number of healthcare customers of the industry as a whole within a designated community for the previous year. An HCO can look at the results of past models to see if they were indeed accurate. This can help the HCO decide if a change has occurred in the marketplace and to identify specific types of people who need healthcare services.

30. A: Main leaders in healthcare organizations maintain oversight and communication with multiple departments and large numbers of people. There is a chain of communication that leads to the governing board in an accountability hierarchy, but many healthcare organizations are under a mesh system. This means that one person, who is the supervisor, has communication over many different channels, and the various departments have unique organizational goals that may be different from the main organization's goals. The mesh system leads to the creation of groups within the organization called service lines. Service lines reflect the needs of their specific patients rather than a generic goal. Objective measurements are used to evaluate service lines and if a service line is not functioning properly, it can be replaced. Service lines understand how easy they can be replaced and in return, function better to avoid it.

31. B: There are three types of prevention of illnesses: primary, secondary, and tertiary. When a shot is given to stop a person from getting sick or any action is taken to avoid an illness, primary prevention is applied. Once an illness has already been established in a patient, secondary prevention is used to lower the negative effects caused by the disease. In order to stop a sickness from happening again or to avoid unnecessary side effects of the disease, tertiary prevention techniques are followed.

32. C: By applying a decision model in the process of determining the best medical course of treatment, the patient can feel secure that whatever treatment is used will be beneficial and necessary. The patient can also feel secure that the doctor has not just based his or her treatment on a test, but rather has applied logic and weighed options before deciding the best course of action. Applying a decision model ensures that the physical and monetary price of a medical procedure is completely necessary for proper treatment. Many times there is more than one way to treat an illness, but applying the decision model assures that the best treatment is chosen. Applying a decision model in the beginning will avoid unnecessary time being wasted on incorrect treatments.

33. D: Clinical expectations are standards for what resources will be required in completion of a medical procedure or patient care. These standards are set and accepted by the medical profession as a whole so patients, insurance providers, and physicians all know in advance what they will need to complete a patient's treatment. Clinical expectations are part of the following three groups: functional protocols, patient care plans, and patient management protocols. Healthcare provider's development is part of the continuous improvement process. Healthcare providers should be encouraged to take a proactive role in determining new and fresh ways of maintaining good clinical performance. Protocols that are established by profession and accepted by a healthcare organization as a whole are called patient management protocols. The goal of using patient management protocols is successful treatment which is measurable, based on the results of using clinical practice guidelines.

34. A: Strategies must be established for a healthcare organization (HCO) to reach the population they service when it comes to leading healthier lifestyles to avoid sicknesses. The goal of the HCO is not to see people in the community for preventable illnesses. By using a decision theory model, the HCO weighs the price of care for an illness against the expenses used to help the person avoid the illness. The HCO looks for ways to provide the community with services to prevent illnesses that make the most financial sense to the organization and that can affect the largest number of people--a process known as optimization of preventive activity.

35. C: Doctors are evaluated based on a system called privileging. The goal of privileging and credentialing is to ensure physicians are qualified to provide medical care. Once qualified, the physician can make medical decisions and provide service to patients. The bylaws of the privileging agreement were set forth by doctors who agreed upon guidelines that all doctors must follow. The physician organization through the bylaws determines standards for care, salary, and other requirements that can be legally upheld if a source of conflict arises. Once a doctor decides to become a part of a physician organization, they are rewarded with privileges as detailed in the privileging agreement.

36. B: Healthcare organizations use a conceptual planning model to determine the number of physicians required. The model multiplies the number of people in the community who will potentially have a medical problem by the number of illnesses or treatments and divides that number by number of treatments completed in the previous year. To determine how many potential doctors need to be hired, a model

is used that takes the previous problem's solution or the number of doctors required and subtracts how many doctors are already working for, and will continue to work for the HCO. The physician recruitment plan requires the HCO to estimate how many people will need specific types of care, how many and how much care their current physicians will provide, and what specialty physicians will be needed to provide patient care.

37. B: Most healthcare organizations (HCOs) have the resources and thus the responsibility to oversee the population it services, to discover areas where more healthcare services are needed, to ensure people are happy with services received, to ensure excellent care is provided, and to correct any areas that are lacking in excellence. This ensures that the HCO is meeting the needs of the population it serves and can make alterations to the services it provides to meet the needs of the community. The HCO has to gather a great deal of information to get accurate and complete data so that it can determine how comprehensive its services are compared to services in other comparable market areas. The Behavioral Risk Factor Surveillance Survey can be accessed to find out state-wide healthcare information which the HCO can use to compare itself against. The goal is not so one HCO can compete against another. The goal of the information is to make all HCOs better for the community.

38. D: The financial management portion of a healthcare organization (HCO) is responsible for locating and tracking any financial dealing that has bearing upon the HCO--which is called transaction accounting. There are many transactions that affect an HCO financially, including employees, furniture for a waiting room, and technology. Every item has a cost and transaction accounting keeps track of every item and cost. Most paper money is collected by an HCO when employees are providing medical assistance, or service to patients and their loved ones. The people working for the HCO and the necessary equipment bought that cannot be sold make up resource transactions--which are also tracked in transaction accounting. The information is input and displayed in cost ledgers. If the transaction occurs within the HCO, it is referred to as a general ledger transaction.

39. B: Part of financial planning for a healthcare organization (HCO) includes the creation of a long range financial plan (LRFP). The strategic plan is analyzed to determine how much money will be brought into the HCO and how much money will be output, which is detailed in the LRFP. Large loans are typically thirty years long and must be factored into financial planning. Ratio analysis is used to compare how much money or capital is leaving the HCO versus how much is coming into the

HCO. Ratio analysis is used to determine if the interest paid and other fees related to borrowing from an outside source is worth it, areas where savings can be found and made, how much actual money is needed to pay off people who the HCO owes money to, and to determine if the consequences of any decisions dealing with money are worth the potential consequences.

40. C: Healthcare organizations (HCOs) are increasingly removing smaller branches and adding them and/or other businesses to the main HCO. If there is more than one healthcare facility in a city, they will often come together to form one large HCO, or join together but function as separate units. Healthcare facilities in several different locations servicing a variety of populations have come together to form large HCOs. These multi-corporate HCOs combine assets, which gives them more of an opportunity to raise money for expansion. The forming of a large corporation or the acquisition of other businesses can be short-term and used to achieve a specific goal. The main HCO can give money to the smaller branch it buys to help better their investments. The HCO can buy a business offering a specific type of service for its benefit. For example, if an HCO needs someone to process lab tests, it can purchase a lab testing company with which it can negotiate a fair price, but also ensure that the lab test company is providing excellent service.

41. C: The Human Resources department creates a workforce plan which is used to determine how many people are needed to work in each department of the healthcare organization (HCO). Human Resources factors in how many people are employed and will continue to be employed for the period of time the workforce plan is created for. The salaries and other compensation for employees should be projected in the workforce plan. If there are known areas where salary or other benefits will change, these should be detailed in the workforce plan. Human Resources must communicate with the various department managers to get information required for the plan. As the organization changes, so should the plan and it therefore requires consistent evaluation. If the plan uncovers a need for new employees or a need for the retention of employees, Human Resources develops strategies to cover the needs.

42. B: Sometimes an employee has an issue or problem that he or she thinks should be investigated. Many healthcare organizations have an ombudsman office to which Human Resources can refer the employee. A representative from the ombudsman office will act as an intermediary to represent the employee in front of the necessary parties. The goal is to diffuse the situation. If this is not possible, and the employee is represented by a union, he can file a formal grievance which can result in the union

bringing legal action against the HCO. Managers should know how to handle the grievance process to avoid the escalation to a lawsuit. Supervisors should keep a well-written account of the problem and look into the problem fairly. Human Resources should try to come up with compromise when available. Even if the employee is not represented by a union, his or her problems matter and Human Resources should take all complaints seriously.

43. C: Many healthcare organizations (HCOs) encourage the use of transformational management. The goal of this type of management is to help employees get better through training and encouragement, rather than through discipline and reprimand. HCOs should train supervisors on strategies that will help them implement transformational management strategies. Many managers are trained to use punitive measures to get what they want from employees, so the transformational style may be new. Management should be well versed in the HCO's principles so it can communicate those principles effectively and clearly to the employees. Managers are responsible for looking at their departments and finding areas that are in need of improvement.

44. D: Healthcare organizations are large and must have space available for the many units contained in their facility. The healthcare buildings must be cleaned and maintained. The food service areas and waiting rooms also must be maintained. The facility maintenance of an HCO is known as a plant system. Part of the responsibility of leadership of the plant system is to use the space within the HCO in the best way possible to provide safety, convenience and aesthetic appeal. When people visiting the healthcare facility feel secure and comfortable, they get better faster. If the HCO looks better, more people will want to visit, so putting money into the design aspects of the HCO is worthwhile. Medical equipment is necessary in an HCO so the design of the HCO must reflect the placement of these necessary items. Some departments of the HCO require more room, which must be provided for in the design of the HCO.

45. A: Consultants, whether internal or external, should be used strategically. The task that is given to the consultants should be well-defined and stated so there is little room for misunderstanding. The more information the consultant has about the area of concern, the better job he or she can do in fixing the problem. If the problem can be fixed by people already employed by the healthcare organization, it should be. Consultants who are experts about the specific problem should be used and if an expert cannot be found, gaining a second or third opinion is a good strategy. The consultants should not be left to work at their own pace and

discretion. The HCO should maintain oversight and make sure the consultants are meeting expectations. There should be clearly defined avenues of communication for the consultants so they can work quickly and efficiently.

46. D: A healthcare organization (HCO) must employ various strategies to determine the needs and wants of its customers so it can develop a marketing strategy that reaches the appropriate people with an appropriate message. Formal surveys are used to question any group of people, from patients to employees, to uncover areas that they want changed or addressed. The HCO can use the information to develop their goals specifically for a group's preference. To gain more information, the HCO can gather small groups of people from a specific market group into a focus group to learn even more about the specific needs of a group of customers. The HCO can identify problem areas by maintaining monitors in the facility. Monitors can be comment cards for employees or customers to fill out, or the requirement of written incident reports when anything goes awry within the HCO. Finally, the HCO will require its supervisors to ask questions and listen to employees and customers.
47. B: The roles of nurses in the healthcare industry are diverse, but overall nurses are meant to provide patients with extended quality care. The American Nurses Association (ANA) has set forth what type of characteristics nurses should possess, beginning with the fact that nurses are meant to develop interactions with patients that help the patient feel better emotionally and physically. People are different and will react differently to health problems and nurses should be able to respond appropriately. The nurse should be able to provide healthcare based on medical knowledge as well as the unique situation of each patient. The nurse should be able to use education and apply it in medical situations to figure out what is wrong with a patient and administer appropriate care. A nurse should be part of some type of continuous education program. The nurse should be an advocate for the population as a whole.

48. A: Nurses create unique patient care plans which respond to the needs and symptoms of the individual patient while following set protocols whenever possible. Sometimes a patient's illness cannot be treated based solely on protocol and the nurse must adapt the protocol in those cases. The nurse must assess the patient based on medical history and by listening to input from the people caring for the patient. Most patients are not cared for by just one doctor, so the nurse should communicate with all of the patient's doctors to determine the best course of treatment for the patient. The care plan needs to include communication with the patient's family on what circumstances the patient will be faced with post-hospital treatment and take into account any special needs. The nurse should also evaluate

the financial status and needs of the patient and how treatment will affect the patient's finances. The patient care plan should have a discharge plan which details when the patient will leave the healthcare facility.

49. D: The people in charge of assignments look at the nursing schedule and make manual adjustments based on needs of the hospital and problems with staff, including unforeseen circumstances like when personnel calls in sick. Nurses who are overworked because there are staffing problems are generally unhappy with their work environment. Part of a quality healthcare organization includes keeping employees happy, so staffing problems should be met with an increased staff whenever possible. If there is a need for more staff in one department that can be fulfilled by another department that has few patients, nurses can move over to cover the need. Many staffing systems can provide this service and can recognize the best placement of patients based on their medical needs and staffing available. If all else fails, there are groups of nurses who have the ability to work in many areas who can be called upon in a time of need. Patient-scheduling systems keep the schedules of patients and can therefore track problems or inadequacies in the treatment of patients in a timely manner.

50. B: For clinical support services (CSSs) to be effective, they must be evaluated and measured for quality. A major area of quality for CSSs is technical quality. If sloppy work is completed or the employees are insufficiently trained to do their job correctly, technical quality is not achieved. A CSS expert should be well-trained and have a formal education to backup his or her training. CSS experts require high salaries so they are typically placed in managerial roles over people with an informal education. The CSS experts should attend ongoing training, which should include tools to overcome professional disagreements between experts that sometimes arise. The CSS experts should also receive special training on how to oversee the nonprofessional staff working beneath them. Protocols are created for CSSs to follow. When the CSS experts and the nonprofessionals receive adequate training regarding accepted protocols, both can provide higher quality healthcare.

# Secret Key #1 – Time is Your Greatest Enemy

## Pace Yourself

Wear a watch to the CPHIMS Test. At the beginning of the test, check the time (or start a chronometer on your watch to count the minutes), and check the time after each passage or every few questions to make sure you are "on schedule." For the computerized test an onscreen clock display will keep track of your remaining time, but it may be easier for you to monitor your pace based on how many minutes have been used, rather than how many minutes remain.

If you find that you are falling behind time during the test, begin skipping difficult questions (unless you know it at a quick glance). Once you catch back up, you can continue working each problem. If you have time at the end, go back then and finish the questions that you left behind.

If you are forced to speed up, do it efficiently. Usually one or more answer choices can be eliminated without too much difficulty. Above all, don't panic. Don't speed up and just begin guessing at random choices. By pacing yourself, and continually monitoring your progress against the clock or your watch, you will always know exactly how far ahead or behind you are with your available time. If you find that you are one minute behind on the test, don't skip one question without spending any time on it, just to catch back up. Spend perhaps 45 seconds on the question and after four questions, you will have caught back up more gradually. Once you catch back up, you can continue working each problem at your normal pace.

Furthermore, don't dwell on the problems that you were rushed on. If a problem was taking up too much time and you made a hurried guess, it must be difficult. The difficult questions are the ones you are most likely to miss anyway, so it isn't a big loss. It is better to end with more time than you need than to run out of time. You can always go back and work the problems that you skipped. If you have time left over, as you review the skipped questions, start at the earliest skipped question, spend at most another minute, and then move on to the next skipped question.

Lastly, sometimes it is beneficial to slow down if you are constantly getting ahead of time. You are always more likely to catch a careless mistake by working more slowly than quickly, and among very high-scoring test takers (those who are likely to have lots of time left over), careless errors affect the score more than mastery of material.

# Secret Key #2 – Guessing is not Guesswork

You probably know that guessing is a good idea on the CPHIMS test- unlike other standardized tests, there is no penalty for getting a wrong answer. Even if you have no idea about a question, you still have a 20-25% chance of getting it right.

Most test takers do not understand the impact that proper guessing can have on their score. Unless you score extremely high, guessing will significantly contribute to your final score.

## Monkeys Take the CPHIMS

What most test takers don't realize is that to insure that 20-25% chance, you have to guess randomly. If you put 20 monkeys in a room to take this test, assuming they answered once per question and behaved themselves, on average they would get 20-25% of the questions correct. Put 20 test takers in the room, and the average will be much lower among guessed questions. Why?

1. This test intentionally writes deceptive answer choices that "look" right. A student has no idea about a question, so picks the "best looking" answer, which is often wrong. The monkey has no idea what looks good and what doesn't, so will consistently be lucky about 20-25% of the time.
2. Test takers will eliminate answer choices from the guessing pool based on a hunch or intuition. Simple but correct answers often get excluded, leaving a 0% chance of being correct. The monkey has no clue, and often gets lucky with the best choice.

This is why the process of elimination endorsed by most test courses is flawed and detrimental to your performance- students don't guess, they make an ignorant stab in the dark that is usually worse than random.

## Success Strategy

Let me introduce one of the most valuable ideas of this course- the $5 challenge:

*You only mark your "best guess" if you are willing to bet $5 on it.*
*You only eliminate choices from guessing if you are willing to bet $5 on it.*

Why $5? Five dollars is an amount of money that is small yet not insignificant, and can really add up fast (20 questions could cost you $100). Likewise, each answer choice on one question of the CPHIMS will have a small impact on your overall score, but it can really add up to a lot of points in the end.

The process of elimination IS valuable. The following shows your chance of guessing it right:

| If you eliminate this many choices: | 0 | 1 | 2 | 3 | 4 |
|---|---|---|---|---|---|
| Chance of getting it correct | 20% | 25% | 33% | 50% | 100% |

However, if you accidentally eliminate the right answer or go on a hunch for an incorrect answer, your chances drop dramatically: to 0%. By guessing among all the answer choices, you are GUARANTEED to have a shot at the right answer.

That's why the $5 test is so valuable- if you give up the advantage and safety of a pure guess, it had better be worth the risk.

What we still haven't covered is how to be sure that whatever guess you make is truly random. Here's the easiest way:

*Always pick the first answer choice among those remaining.*

Such a technique means that you have decided, **before you see a single test question**, exactly how you are going to guess- and since the order of choices tells you nothing about which one is correct, this guessing technique is perfectly random.

# Secret Key #3 – Practice Smarter, Not Harder

Many test takers delay the test preparation process because they dread the awful amounts of practice time they think necessary to succeed on the test. We have refined an effective method that will take you only a fraction of the time.

There are a number of "obstacles" in your way on the CPHIMS test. Among these are answering questions, finishing in time, and mastering test-taking strategies. All must be executed on the day of the test at peak performance, or your score will suffer. The CPHIMS is a mental marathon that has a large impact on your future.

Just like a marathon runner, it is important to work your way up to the full challenge. So first you just worry about questions, and then time, and finally strategy:

## Success Strategy

1. Find a good source for CPHIMS practice tests. You will need at least 2 practice tests.
2. If you are willing to make a larger time investment (or if you want to really "learn" the material, a time consuming but ultimately valuable endeavor), consider buying one of the better study guides on the market.
3. Take a practice test with no time constraints, with all study helps "open book." Take your time with questions and focus on applying the strategies.
4. Take a final practice test with no open material and time limits.

If you have time to take more practice tests, just repeat step 4. By gradually exposing yourself to the full rigors of the test environment, you will condition your mind to the stress of test day and maximize your success.

## Secret Key #4 – Prepare, Don't Procrastinate

Let me state an obvious fact: if you take the CPHIMS exam three times, you will get three different scores. This is due to the way you feel on test day, the level of preparedness you have, and, despite CPHIMS exam's claims to the contrary, some tests WILL be easier for you than others.

Since your success will largely depend on your score, you should maximize your chances of success. In order to maximize the likelihood of success, you've got to prepare in advance. This means taking practice tests and spending time learning the information and test taking strategies you will need to succeed.

Since you have to pay a registration fee each time you take the CPHIMS exam, don't take it as a "practice" test. Feel free to take sample tests on your own, but when you go to take the CPHIMS exam, be prepared, be focused, and do your best the first time!

# Secret Key #5 – Test Yourself

Everyone knows that time is money. There is no need to spend too much of your time or too little of your time preparing for the CPHIMS exam. You should only spend as much of your precious time preparing as is necessary for you to pass it.

## Success Strategy

Once you have taken a practice test under real conditions of time constraints, then you will know if you are ready for the test or not.

If you have scored extremely high the first time that you take the practice test, then there is not much point in spending countless hours studying. You are already there.

Benchmark your abilities by retaking practice tests and seeing how much you have improved. Once you score high enough to guarantee success, then you are ready.

If you have scored well below where you need, then knuckle down and begin studying in earnest. Check your improvement regularly through the use of practice tests under real conditions. Above all, don't worry, panic, or give up. The key is perseverance!

Then, when you go to take the CPHIMS exam, remain confident and remember how well you did on the practice tests. If you can score high enough on a practice test, then you can do the same on the real thing.

# General Strategies

The most important thing you can do is to ignore your fears and jump into the test immediately- do not be overwhelmed by any strange-sounding terms. You have to jump into the test like jumping into a pool- all at once is the easiest way.

**Make Predictions**

As you read and understand the question, try to guess what the answer will be. Remember that several of the answer choices are wrong, and once you begin reading them, your mind will immediately become cluttered with answer choices designed to throw you off. Your mind is typically the most focused immediately after you have read the question and digested its contents. If you can, try to predict what the correct answer will be. You may be surprised at what you can predict.

Quickly scan the choices and see if your prediction is in the listed answer choices. If it is, then you can be quite confident that you have the right answer. It still won't hurt to check the other answer choices, but most of the time, you've got it!

**Answer the Question**

It may seem obvious to only pick answer choices that answer the question, but the test writers can create some excellent answer choices that are wrong. Don't pick an answer just because it sounds right, or you believe it to be true. It MUST answer the question. Once you've made your selection, always go back and check it against the question and make sure that you didn't misread the question, and the answer choice does answer the question posed.

**Benchmark**

After you read the first answer choice, decide if you think it sounds correct or not. If it doesn't, move on to the next answer choice. If it does, mentally mark that answer choice. This doesn't mean that you've definitely selected it as your answer choice, it just means that it's the best you've seen thus far. Go ahead and read the next choice. If the next choice is worse than the one you've already selected, keep going to the next answer choice. If the next choice is better than the choice you've already selected, mentally mark the new answer choice as your best guess.

The first answer choice that you select becomes your standard. Every other answer choice must be benchmarked against that standard. That choice is correct until proven otherwise by another answer choice beating it out. Once you've decided that no other answer choice seems as good, do one final check to ensure that your answer choice answers the question posed.

**Valid Information**

Don't discount any of the information provided in the question. Every piece of information may be necessary to determine the correct answer. None of the information in the question is there to throw you off (while the answer choices will certainly have information to throw you off). If two seemingly unrelated topics are discussed, don't ignore either. You can be confident there is a relationship, or it wouldn't be included in the question, and you are probably going to have to determine what is that relationship to find the answer.

**Avoid "Fact Traps"**

Don't get distracted by a choice that is factually true. Your search is for the answer that answers the question. Stay focused and don't fall for an answer that is true but incorrect. Always go back to the question and make sure you're choosing an answer that actually answers the question and is not just a true statement. An answer can be factually correct, but it MUST answer the question asked. Additionally, two answers can both be seemingly correct, so be sure to read all of the answer choices, and make sure that you get the one that BEST answers the question.

**Milk the Question**

Some of the questions may throw you completely off. They might deal with a subject you have not been exposed to, or one that you haven't reviewed in years. While your lack of knowledge about the subject will be a hindrance, the question itself can give you many clues that will help you find the correct answer. Read the question carefully and look for clues. Watch particularly for adjectives and nouns describing difficult terms or words that you don't recognize. Regardless of if you completely understand a word or not, replacing it with a synonym either provided or one you more familiar with may help you to understand what the questions are asking. Rather than wracking your mind about specific detailed information concerning a difficult term or word, try to use mental substitutes that are easier to understand.

### The Trap of Familiarity

Don't just choose a word because you recognize it. On difficult questions, you may not recognize a number of words in the answer choices. The test writers don't put "make-believe" words on the test; so don't think that just because you only recognize all the words in one answer choice means that answer choice must be correct. If you only recognize words in one answer choice, then focus on that one. Is it correct? Try your best to determine if it is correct. If it is, that is great, but if it doesn't, eliminate it. Each word and answer choice you eliminate increases your chances of getting the question correct, even if you then have to guess among the unfamiliar choices.

### Eliminate Answers

Eliminate choices as soon as you realize they are wrong. But be careful! Make sure you consider all of the possible answer choices. Just because one appears right, doesn't mean that the next one won't be even better! The test writers will usually put more than one good answer choice for every question, so read all of them. Don't worry if you are stuck between two that seem right. By getting down to just two remaining possible choices, your odds are now 50/50. Rather than wasting too much time, play the odds. You are guessing, but guessing wisely, because you've been able to knock out some of the answer choices that you know are wrong. If you are eliminating choices and realize that the last answer choice you are left with is also obviously wrong, don't panic. Start over and consider each choice again. There may easily be something that you missed the first time and will realize on the second pass.

### Tough Questions

If you are stumped on a problem or it appears too hard or too difficult, don't waste time. Move on! Remember though, if you can quickly check for obviously incorrect answer choices, your chances of guessing correctly are greatly improved. Before you completely give up, at least try to knock out a couple of possible answers. Eliminate what you can and then guess at the remaining answer choices before moving on.

### Brainstorm

If you get stuck on a difficult question, spend a few seconds quickly brainstorming. Run through the complete list of possible answer choices. Look at each choice and ask yourself, "Could this answer the question satisfactorily?" Go through each answer choice and consider it independently of the other. By systematically going through all possibilities, you may find something that you would otherwise overlook. Remember that when you get stuck, it's important to try to keep moving.

## Read Carefully

Understand the problem. Read the question and answer choices carefully. Don't miss the question because you misread the terms. You have plenty of time to read each question thoroughly and make sure you understand what is being asked. Yet a happy medium must be attained, so don't waste too much time. You must read carefully, but efficiently.

## Face Value

When in doubt, use common sense. Always accept the situation in the problem at face value. Don't read too much into it. These problems will not require you to make huge leaps of logic. The test writers aren't trying to throw you off with a cheap trick. If you have to go beyond creativity and make a leap of logic in order to have an answer choice answer the question, then you should look at the other answer choices. Don't overcomplicate the problem by creating theoretical relationships or explanations that will warp time or space. These are normal problems rooted in reality. It's just that the applicable relationship or explanation may not be readily apparent and you have to figure things out. Use your common sense to interpret anything that isn't clear.

## Prefixes

If you're having trouble with a word in the question or answer choices, try dissecting it. Take advantage of every clue that the word might include. Prefixes and suffixes can be a huge help. Usually they allow you to determine a basic meaning. Pre- means before, post- means after, pro - is positive, de- is negative. From these prefixes and suffixes, you can get an idea of the general meaning of the word and try to put it into context. Beware though of any traps. Just because con is the opposite of pro, doesn't necessarily mean congress is the opposite of progress!

## Hedge Phrases

Watch out for critical "hedge" phrases, such as likely, may, can, will often, sometimes, often, almost, mostly, usually, generally, rarely, sometimes. Question writers insert these hedge phrases to cover every possibility. Often an answer choice will be wrong simply because it leaves no room for exception. Avoid answer choices that have definitive words like "exactly," and "always".

**Switchback Words**

Stay alert for "switchbacks". These are the words and phrases frequently used to alert you to shifts in thought. The most common switchback word is "but". Others include although, however, nevertheless, on the other hand, even though, while, in spite of, despite, regardless of.

**New Information**

Correct answer choices will rarely have completely new information included. Answer choices typically are straightforward reflections of the material asked about and will directly relate to the question. If a new piece of information is included in an answer choice that doesn't even seem to relate to the topic being asked about, then that answer choice is likely incorrect. All of the information needed to answer the question is usually provided for you, and so you should not have to make guesses that are unsupported or choose answer choices that require unknown information that cannot be reasoned on its own.

**Time Management**

On technical questions, don't get lost on the technical terms. Don't spend too much time on any one question. If you don't know what a term means, then since you don't have a dictionary, odds are you aren't going to get much further. You should immediately recognize terms as whether or not you know them. If you don't, work with the other clues that you have, the other answer choices and terms provided, but don't waste too much time trying to figure out a difficult term.

**Contextual Clues**

Look for contextual clues. An answer can be right but not correct. The contextual clues will help you find the answer that is most right and is correct. Understand the context in which a phrase or statement is made. This will help you make important distinctions.

**Don't Panic**

Panicking will not answer any questions for you. Therefore, it isn't helpful. When you first see the question, if your mind goes blank, take a deep breath. Force yourself to mechanically go through the steps of solving the problem and using the strategies you've learned.

**Pace Yourself**

Don't get clock fever. It's easy to be overwhelmed when you're looking at a page full of questions, your mind is full of random thoughts and feeling confused, and the clock is ticking down faster than you would like. Calm down and maintain the pace that you have set for yourself. As long as you are on track by monitoring your pace, you are guaranteed to have enough time for yourself. When you get to the last few minutes of the test, it may seem like you won't have enough time left, but if you only have as many questions as you should have left at that point, then you're right on track!

**Answer Selection**

The best way to pick an answer choice is to eliminate all of those that are wrong, until only one is left and confirm that is the correct answer. Sometimes though, an answer choice may immediately look right. Be careful! Take a second to make sure that the other choices are not equally obvious. Don't make a hasty mistake. There are only two times that you should stop before checking other answers. First is when you are positive that the answer choice you have selected is correct. Second is when time is almost out and you have to make a quick guess!

**Check Your Work**

Since you will probably not know every term listed and the answer to every question, it is important that you get credit for the ones that you do know. Don't miss any questions through careless mistakes. If at all possible, try to take a second to look back over your answer selection and make sure you've selected the correct answer choice and haven't made a costly careless mistake (such as marking an answer choice that you didn't mean to mark). This quick double check should more than pay for itself in caught mistakes for the time it costs.

**Beware of Directly Quoted Answers**

Sometimes an answer choice will repeat word for word a portion of the question or reference section. However, beware of such exact duplication – it may be a trap! More than likely, the correct choice will paraphrase or summarize a point, rather than being exactly the same wording.

**Slang**

Scientific sounding answers are better than slang ones. An answer choice that begins "To compare the outcomes…" is much more likely to be correct than one that begins "Because some people insisted…"

**Extreme Statements**

Avoid wild answers that throw out highly controversial ideas that are proclaimed as established fact. An answer choice that states the "process should be used in certain situations, if…" is much more likely to be correct than one that states the "process should be discontinued completely." The first is a calm rational statement and doesn't even make a definitive, uncompromising stance, using a hedge word "if" to provide wiggle room, whereas the second choice is a radical idea and far more extreme.

**Answer Choice Families**

When you have two or more answer choices that are direct opposites or parallels, one of them is usually the correct answer. For instance, if one answer choice states "x increases" and another answer choice states "x decreases" or "y increases," then those two or three answer choices are very similar in construction and fall into the same family of answer choices. A family of answer choices is when two or three answer choices are very similar in construction, and yet often have a directly opposite meaning. Usually the correct answer choice will be in that family of answer choices. The "odd man out" or answer choice that doesn't seem to fit the parallel construction of the other answer choices is more likely to be incorrect.

# Special Report: Additional Bonus Material

Due to our efforts to try to keep this book to a manageable length, we've created a link that will give you access to all of your additional bonus material.

Please visit http://www.mometrix.com/bonus948/cphims to access the information.